Bodies and Suffering

This book is a critical response to a range of problems – some theoretical, others empirical – that shape questions surrounding the lived experience of suffering. It explores how moral and ethical questions of personal suffering are experienced, contested, negotiated and institutionalised. *Bodies and Suffering* investigates the moral labour and significance invested in actions to care for others, or in failing to do so. It also explores circumstances – personal, political and social – under which that which is perceived as non-moral becomes moral.

Drawing on case studies and empirical research, *Bodies and Suffering* examines the idea of the suffering body across different cultures and contexts and the experience and treatment of these suffering bodies. The book draws on theories of affect, embodiment, the phenomenology of illness and moralities of care, to produce a nuanced understanding of suffering as being located across the assumed borders of time, space, bodies, persons and things.

Suitable for bioethicists, medical anthropologists, health sociologists and body studies scholars, *Bodies and Suffering* will also be of use on health science courses as essential reading on suffering bodies, mental health and morality and ethics issues.

Ana Dragojlovic is a Lecturer in Gender Studies at the University of Melbourne, Australia.

Alex Broom is Professor of Sociology in the School of Social Sciences, and in the Practical Justice Initiative, UNSW Australia.

Routledge Advances in the Medical Humanities

Bodies and Suffering

Emotions and Relations of Care

Ana Dragojlovic and Alex Broom

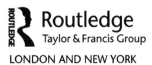

LONDON AND NEW YORK

First published 2018
by Routledge
4 Park Square, Milton Park, Abingdon, Oxon OX14 4RN
605 Third Avenue, New York, NY 10017

First issued in paperback 2023

Routledge is an imprint of the Taylor & Francis Group, an informa business

British Library Cataloguing-in-Publication Data
A catalogue record for this book is available from the British Library

Library of Congress Cataloging-in-Publication Data
Names: Dragojlovic, Ana. | Broom, Alex.
Title: Bodies and suffering : emotions and relations of care /
    Ana Dragojlovic and Alex Broom.
Other titles: Routledge advances in the medical humanities.
Description: Abingdon, Oxon ; New York, N : Routledge, 2017. |
Series: Routledge advances in the medical humanities |
    Includes bibliographical references and index.
Identifiers: LCCN 2017005739| ISBN 9781138885264 (hardback) |
    ISBN 9781315715568 (ebook)
Subjects: | MESH: Patient Care | Pain | Stress, Psychological |
    Bioethical Issues
Classification: LCC RA399.A1 | NLM W 84.1 | DDC 362.1068—dc23
LC record available at https://lccn.loc.gov/2017005739

ISBN: 978-0-367-22448-6 (pbk)
ISBN: 978-1-138-88526-4 (hbk)
ISBN: 978-1-315-71556-8 (ebk)

DOI: 10.4324/9781315715568

Typeset in Times New Roman
by Apex CoVantage, LLC

Publisher's Note
The publisher has gone to great lengths to ensure the quality of this reprint but points out that some imperfections in the original copies may be apparent.

Contents

Introduction

Bodies and suffering – affect, emotions and relations of care

Suffering is an inextricable aspect of the human condition. To live is to suffer, in some form, and at some time. Suffering has many layers, moves across people/s, and is thus extraordinarily difficult to define. Suffering is unequally distributed and is embedded in structures of disadvantage and domination. Even the most seemingly straightforward question becomes problematic when examined closely – what is suffering and what does it mean for a person to suffer? Is the experience of suffering culturally relative – is it contingent on the individual's perspective – and can we meaningfully compare experiences? Consider the context of a person in Haiti living in abject poverty, or the Syrian wounded and displaced in Aleppo, and compare them with an Australian 'middle-class' person who is dying; or, as we do in the following chapters, people suffering from intergenerational distress caused by historical violence. Whilst they *may* all *consider themselves* and *be considered* to be suffering, what does it mean 'to suffer' across these vastly different contexts, bodies and persons? What links them, what connects them, if anything? This cascading complexity is further enhanced when we consider, for example, how relevant external conditions are versus the inner world of the person in understanding suffering. Does it matter what a person's life, a moment in time, or a particular lived experience looks like (externally) versus feels like? Suffering as a concept challenges our understandings of things, requiring consideration of a series of entrenched dialectics around concreteness versus subjectivities, physicality versus emotionality, externality versus internality. Moreover, in writing and thinking about suffering, who, if anyone, should be able to speak to peoples' experiences – to embark on a process of characterising or narrating a person's experience of suffering? The question of suffering cannot be examined without consideration of who suffers, for what reasons, and to what end (Kleinman, 1988). This requires recognition of suffering as a lived experience that is embedded in political, economic and cultural contexts, and as a product of the organisation of modern society/ies (Bourdieu, 1999; Cohen, 2013). In *Bodies and Suffering*, we seek to shed light on different aspects of these questions and dilemmas, moving back and forward from the particularities of case studies, to the broader theoretical dimensions of suffering. We will weave together emerging theoretical concerns, with the unruliness of specific sites of suffering, across cultures, peoples and groups.

Many of the questions posed above in regards to suffering and the human condition, have been raised across many different academic disciplines over the course of the last few centuries (Kleinman et al., 1997). Philosophers, for instance, have tended to situate suffering within the frame of ethics and moralities (Held, 1995, 2005; Larrabee, 1993); social science scholars have often engaged in suffering in terms of justice and human rights (Bubeck, 1995); anthropologists/development studies scholars have often focused on the lived experience, structural violence and social suffering (Farmer, 1996; Goodin, 1985; Kleinman et al., 1997); and gender studies scholars have focused on forms of cultural/ideological violence and the politics and practices of (gendered) domination (Marecek, 2006). There are many more interpretive traditions which have captured the gendered, political, cultural, economic and philosophical facets of suffering in social life (Bourdieu, 1999; Cohen, 2013; Kleinman, 1992). We will explore several of these traditions in this book. What they share, as does our analysis, is a recognition that in the context of neoliberalism, suffering is much more than an individual experience, and yet is revealed only through explorations of the individual's experience (Bauman, 2013). By 'neoliberalism', we are referring to the major changes on economic, political and social arrangements that begun following the signing of the North American Free Trade Agreement in 1994. These changes are characterised by changing market relations, changing the role of the state and an increasing emphasis on individual responsibility. Scholars have argued that the extension of competitive markets into all spheres of life – the economy, politics, education, health, and so forth – is the main characteristic of neoliberalism (Bourdieu, 1999; Davies, 2012; Harvey, 2005; Springer et al., 2016). In this book, we argue that neoliberalism is a messy, diffuse set of assemblages of suffering. Suffering is thus at once a lived experience, an affective relation, and a cultural, economic and political assemblage. Suffering is frequently an outcome of the (often unfulfilled) 'contract' between the modern nation state and individual (Rousseau, 1920). Some facets of suffering are inevitable, while others are political and economic choices – considered a 'reasonable' price to pay for the nation's structural/economic success (Cohen, 2013). Whilst many states fail to address it or live up to their 'end of the bargain', as it were, it is nonetheless true that suffering is a constitutive feature of the current political milieu (at least in most democratic nations, and however diverse across contexts) (Bauman, 2013). And, the (regular) failures of modern states to fulfil this social contract, has been fertile ground for social scientists (Farmer, 1996). Each tradition has added new understandings, detailing often dramatic and tragic events across the world (Das et al., 2000; Kleinman et al., 1997), endeavouring to provide measures of healing and to foster public recognition for those who have endured extreme suffering. Our aim here is to embed suffering in the organisation of societies and the current (and previous) global world order, as well as in the minutia of the everyday (Farmer, 1996).

Bodies and suffering

In *Bodies and Suffering*, we build on the existing scholarship on suffering, taking into account the materiality and physicality of the body as much as the disciplining effect of discourse and social narratives (Latimer, 2008; Munro & Belova, 2008). Focusing our analysis on experiences of illness, the end of life, different forms of distress cause by mobility and historical violence, we approach human suffering as affective assemblages of bodies (human and non-human), discourses, practices, and performances and their complex relationality. Positioning our work within critical body theory, we argue that suffering, as affective assemblages, are historically, socially, culturally, politically, economically and morally situated. Based on rich anthropological and sociological empirical research, this book does not seek methodological integration (more on this below) but rather engages different methodologies in order to highlight the fundamental relationality of the suffering assemblage. We contribute to scholarship that argues for a cessation of Cartesian dualism, which dominates various scholarly disciplines, including our fields of anthropology and sociology. Through the analysis of a plethora of empirical material, we seek to obscure and further challenge the problematic split between the mind and the body, and focus on destabilising the distinction between binary notions of health and illness, carers and cared for. Our analysis demonstrates the importance of the embodied, affective and intersubjective, and related ontological conditions.

In particular, we aim to build on, and contribute to the growing field of body studies that has been emerging within the fields of sociology, anthropology and cultural theory (e.g. Shilling, 2003; Blackman, 2008, 2012; Shildrick & Steinberg, 2015). Our approach is informed by earlier studies of embodiment that problematised the distinctions between individual and social, biological and cultural, the mind and the body (Csordas, 1994). While immensely important, such scholarship focused predominantly on the human subject, while neglecting to take into account the importance of non-human bodies and technologies. We study body and embodiment as a process of becoming, and explore how suffering bodies relate to the world. As such, our approach is inspired by and critical of the 'affective turn' (e.g. Ahmed, 2004 a, b; Blackman, 2012; Brennan, 2004; Seigworth & Gregg, 2010; Leys, 2011a, b; Massumi, 2002; Navaro-Yashin, 2012; Thrift, 2008; Wetherell, 2012) in contemporary cultural analyses and the related 'new materialism' (e.g. Braidotti, 2013; Coole & Frost, 2010) that has emerged in the wake of poststructuralism, as a corrective to the 'discursive' and 'linguistic' focus of the 1970s and 1980s. The latter has been criticised for giving primacy to language and discourse over matter and visceral, lived experiences of the body.

Suffering as affective assemblage

This book is about emotive and affective relations of care. In framing our approach this way, we are proposing a reconceptualisation of suffering that extends beyond the human subject to study how suffering bodies affectively relate to human and non-human, self and the other. Here, we follow Deleuze and Guattari, for whom assemblages include elements such as human bodies, matter and things, but also 'semiotic systems' that include 'discourses, words, 'meanings' and noncorporeal relations that link signifiers with effect' (Wise, 2005, p. 80). Deleuze and Guattari argue that the 'functioning of the assemblage can be explained only if one takes it apart to examine both the elements that make it up and the nature of the linkages' (Deleuze & Guattari, 1986, p. 53). As much as we are interested in the various elements of the assemblage and the linkages between them, we are equally engaged in the exploration of *what assemblages do* (Deleuze & Guattari, 1987, p. 257).

Assemblages are produced and shaped by affects. In contemporary scholarship, affect has been described as autonomous, non-representational, trans-subjective, immaterial, or non-conscious (Massumi, 2002; Thrift, 2008; Blackman & Venn, 2010; Seigworth & Gregg, 2010), referring to processes that circulate among bodies (Blackman, 2012; Brennan, 2004) and between bodies and their environments (Navaro-Yashin, 2012). Affect is ambiguous, and there is no originary state from which it begins: 'Affect arises in the midst of *in-between-ness*: in the capacities to act and be acted upon . . . in those intensities that pass body to body' (Seigworth & Gregg, 2010, p. 1). In our analysis, we are not so much interested in what affect *is* but rather what it *does*. As Sara Ahmed persuasively argues, affective dynamics have generative qualities: 'We are moved by things. And in being moved we make things' (2010, p. 33).[1]

It is important to state that, while most affect theorists agree that affects circulate between human and non-human bodies, there are epistemological and ontological disagreements within the 'affect turn' scholarship. This makes it important for us to situate or own approach. The main divergence stems from disagreements about whether affect is pre-individual and pre-subjective, intentional or non-intentional. A prominent group of affect theorists including Brian Massumi (2002), Nigel Thrift (2008) and Patricia Clough (2007) argue for affect as an outside stimulus that hits the body first and as such, is pre-individual and pre-subjective. Our approach to affect builds on the work of Sara Ahmed (2004a, b; 2010), Ruth Leys (2011), Lisa Blackman (2012), Margaret Wetherell (2012), and Yael Navaro-Yashin (2012). This work approaches affect as intensities circulating between human and non-human bodies that are subjectively experienced (see also Dragojlovic, 2015; Knudsen and Stage 2015). Following the lead of Ruth Leys, Lisa Blackman (2012), a historian of science, cautions against the view that affect is only aligned with the non-cognitive. Leys (2011a, b) has offered a nuanced critique of the affect theories within the humanities that insist on a separation of affect from cognition, meaning and interpretation. Examining the work of geographer Nigel Thrift, cultural critic Eric Shouse, political philosopher and social theorist Brian Massumi and political theorist William Connolly, Leys (2011a) contends that, regardless of certain differences in their approaches, all of these scholars theorise affect as prior to and independent from intentions, meanings, beliefs and reason. For these theorists, affects have the intensity and force to influence thinking and judgement, but are simultaneously separate from them. Both Leys (2011a) and Blackman (2012) argue against an ontological commitment to non-intentionality of affect because of the shaky empirical grounds on which the proponents of non-intentionality base their arguments.

Following Lisa Blackman (2012) and Yael Navaro-Yashin (2012), in particular, we argue that while it is important to take into our account affects pre-subjective and non-intentional aspects it is equally important to engage with the subjective experiences of affect and how such experiences are given meaning in specific context. Banishing the subject and the subjective from the theories of affect we might run into a danger of perpetuating dichotomies of mind and body, intentional and non-intentional, cognitive and affective, thus limiting rather than broadening our understanding of the complexities of affect and the affective (and see also Dragojlovic, 2015). Like Ahmed (2004a, b), we use affect almost synonymously with emotions as far as this term does not make a separation between conscious and unconscious, intentional and non-intentional, mind and the body, human and non-human. We also wish to clarify that unlike earlier conceptualisations of emotion, which argue that emotion is determined by culture and norms and primarily expressed through language, we argue that affect relates to intensities that are less shaped, and our understanding of affect does not exclusively focus on the human (see also Navaro-Yashin, 2012).[2]

Instructive for our analysis has been engagement with recent feminist scholarship that, in a special issue of the journal *Body & Society*, debates the shifting grounds for what they call 'biomedical imaginary' by focusing on the analysis of 'estranged bodies' (Shildrick & Steinberg, 2015). Noticing an important absence of engagement with the Deleuzian notion of assemblage in the scholarship about biomedicine, Shildrick and Steinberg noticed an important paradox in biomedical imaginary, according to which an injured body can be repaired to its original wholeness (2015, p. 8). Arguing that human bodies are not singular, stable, or bounded entities, Shildrick and Steinberg cogently argued for the need to engage with Deleuzian analysis in order to approach embodiment as always in process of change and always in relation to human and non-human bodies (animals and machines). Following this line of argument, Lisa Diedrich makes a compelling argument for understanding illness as an assemblage in the same issue of *Body & Society*. Focusing her analysis on the genealogy of the hysteron-epilepsy condition, Diedrich demonstrates how illness is 'made, unmade, and remade in the clinic and narrative' (2015, p. 66). Mobilising the Deluzian notion of assemblage, she argues that, in the case of hysteron-epilepsy condition, illness is composed of an assemblage of diagnosis, bodies, treatments, narratives, practices and discourses (2015, p. 68). Understanding illness as assemblage, Diedrich points to 'twists, turns, ambiguities' (2015, p. 83) of the corporeal, demonstrating the impossibility of a singular, unified self and that embodiment is always in a process of change and becoming. Similarly, we write about suffering as affective assemblages, asserting that they are fundamentally related to human and non-human processes, performances and discourses. As such, we engage in an analysis of *what assemblages do*, in order to highlight the importance of multiple elements and forces of suffering assemblages and to argue for their historical, social, cultural, political, and economic specificities. We explore how affective forces of structural racism and non-normative families affect the economy of marginalization and exclusion, and how in turn those affected by them engage in affective politics by mobilizing politics of negative affect (see Chapters 3 and 4).

Furthermore, in the context of illness, dying and care (both paid and personal), we examine how medical technologies, expert knowledge, prognostic forecasting are part of, actors within, and critical to, experiences of suffering (in relation), and how various affective dimensions (e.g. hope and hopelessness, melancholia and optimism, resilience and wilfulness) are produced through, and in some cases, despite of, these evolving assemblages of illness and care. Chapters 1 and 2 explore the carer's position. Chapter 6 focuses on the lived experiences of affliction, facing mortality, and the affective dimensions of survivorship assemblages. The latter chapter looks specifically at the experiences of cancer patients, particularly those who in the advanced stages of the disease.

Caring relations and being in/with suffering

As noted above, we approach suffering as affective assemblages of which relations of care and caregiving are an inextricable part. Thus, suffering is necessary about care – sometimes lack thereof – whether *in relation to* a partner, family, friend, stranger, community, paid worker, service provider, the state, and so on. As explored in the following chapters, experiences of suffering raise important questions about how one feels in relation to a specific (a family member) and/ or generalised (a government, a community) 'other'. This includes consideration of what caring (or non-caring) relations may or may not offer to 'us' and 'them'. Here we are particularly interested in how such categories becomes compromised or problematized within the lived experience of suffering and care. The presence, absence or particular *form of care*, as experienced, may be critical to the experience of suffering in a person's life world. Suffering is thus deeply intimately enmeshed in evolving, situated and affective relations of care, involving moral, ethical and affective struggles that *being in* and *being with* suffering may induce. Whilst a reductive analysis would outline a discrete sufferer and carer subjective position, a more nuanced analysis, as we pursue in the following chapters, reveals how lines become blurred, with a relational ontology necessary to explore how affective relations are co-produced, move across bodies and persons, and create (and are created by) atmospheres of pain, hope, guilt, resilience, recovery, and persistence. In this sense, any analysis of suffering must be accompanied by an understanding of what constitutes care in neoliberal societies, how it is 'provided' and 'received' and the problematics of such dualisms. Care is, in effect (and in affect), the (somewhat troubled) companion of suffering.

Care-giving, in its many forms and contexts, has a long history and thus so too does the scholarly literature on care. For example, scholarly work on care has sought to unsettle notions of care as imposed (i.e. obligation, structure) or desired/ expressed (i.e. gift, reciprocity); rather positioning caregiving as an assemblage of the relational, normative, discursive and affective relations (Held, 2005; see also Gordon et al., 1996). This has challenged and reconstituted the value of care for the individual (both 'in receipt' and 'providing') rather than positioning it as a responsibility, burden or obligation. This work also articulates the importance of care as a political and civil duty; situating caring as a morally correct disposition towards others and as central to human life (Goodin, 1985; Held, 1995, 2005; Tronto, 1998). This line of inquiry has in turn engaged in the dialectic of care as dependency versus care as a public good (Kittay & Feder, 2002) – a dilemma increasingly acute in the context of economic tightening, individualisation, and, a shrinking welfare and social care sector. Such work raises the problematic of an emerging *freedom from*, rather than a *freedom to*, care (Gordon et al., 1996). Such dynamics are important for understanding the contemporary experience of suffering, but also, how people feel about being cared for (in the context of suffering) but also in their *offerings of care* to those who are suffering.

There is also a gendered, economic and political context to such dynamics of care, whether occurring in the home, community or institution. Care more broadly has been traditionally 'valued privately, romanticised publicly and largely invisible to society' (Gordon et al., 1996, p. viii). This has been recognised within feminist scholarship on care and caregiving, which has positioned caring relations as (traditionally) part of the (often hidden) burden of women's social position and identity (Mol, 2008). Some of the classic work on caring – including that of Finch and Groves (1983) and Larrabee (1993) – interrogated the dilemmas around agency and choice versus gendered obligation in participation in care, the exploitation of women in caregiving, and the complicity of informal caring relations in the perpetuation of gender inequality and barriers to social justice (e.g. Clement, 1996; Gilligan, 1982; Graham, 1991; Poole and Isaacs, 1997; Ungerson, 1983). This work, and others within the field, has raised tensions between meaning and fulfilment versus the imposition of, and assignment to, caring roles (e.g. Bubeck, 1995; Fisher & Tronto, 1990; Tronto, 1993; Twigg & Atkin, 1994; West, 2002). That is, what forms of (often gendered) obligation operate within the context of care for those who suffer, and what moral and normative structures perpetuate such relations (and whose interests these serve, and to what end). In the context of formalised, paid care, the shift to medicalisation (in medicine), professionalisation (in nursing and social care) has somewhat concealed the enduring (affective and gendered) relations of care, even in institutional contexts. As we see in Chapters 1, 2 and 6, suffering is often concealed within the medicalisation of suffering in formalised care contexts, despite being felt in distinctly gendered ways.

Care is, of course, not just an emotion; it has practical facets. As Sara Ahmed (2004a) cogently argued 'emotions do things'. There has also been a focus on disentangling the dimensions of care, including its affective (i.e. loving or other facets/affects of caring) and logistical/physical dimensions (Graham, 1991; Kittay, 1999; Parker, 1993; Ungerson, 1987). Such analysis has inserted complexity into understandings of different sites and spheres of care, in turn illustrating that providing and receiving care is mediated by identity, roles and institutional setting (see, for example, Graham, 1991). This has also involved recognising caring relations as being imbued by power, authority and dependency, highlighting the vulnerability and experiences of suffering for both the care recipient and the carer, as well as the dynamics of physical and/or emotional dependency therein (Kittay, 1999). Work in the field of critical disability studies has emphasized the importance of paying attention to power relations within the relations of care and stressing that care can limit the personal autonomy of care receivers (Williams, 2001). This remains important for understanding the dynamics of caring in the context of human suffering. In the following chapters, we thus seek to reveal the affective elements of care (Bracke et al., 2008; Parker, 1993, Twigg & Atkin, 1994). In doing this, we problematise the valorisation of caregiving, arguing that this itself represents a site of considerable suffering (for carers) and potentially, the 'cared for'.

Whilst *to care for* has traditionally been considered virtuous, despite limited recognition as a social act/relation (particularly for women), to be willing *to receive care* has also been an important dynamic in the landscapes of suffering. What underpins such relations are complex moralities and forms of obligation that circulate around suffering, care and expectations for 'recovery'. This is what we call the *moral economy of caring and affliction*. What do we mean by this? This facet of our work focuses on what it – caring and suffering – requires of its subjects and the potential complicity in the perpetuation of affective distress. Modern medicine provides many examples of the social contract surrounding illness, and the idea that sickness and/or suffering becomes legitimised through a 'proper' medical diagnosis, an agreement regard biophysical pathology, and a mutual understanding of the pathway to health (or wellness). Another way of articulating such dynamics is within a morality of illness, distress and wellness. Here, we seek to unpack the moralities that underpin suffering – how moral and ethical *responses to* suffering (whether 'sufferer' or 'carer') are experienced, contested, negotiated and institutionalised. In the following chapters, we are interested in the *moral labour of care* for others, or indeed, failing to do so, and the (often professional) circumstances whereby that which is perhaps immoral (i.e. distanced, dissociated, dis-engaged) becomes accepted as normal.

In exploring the moral components of suffering and caring, we will utilise contemporary work on the politics of optimism (Berlant, 2011) and wilfulness (Ahmed, 2014), to explore how certain scripts, acts and assemblages of care and recovery are valorised, for what purpose, and to what end? We will ask whether and how suffering is part of this broader moral economy, how the individual experiences may reflect the wider cultural 'pressures' *at work*, and how subjects are governed in suffering. In particular, we will explore how such things as taboo, shame, and obligation are utilised to encourage certain pathways; how they form and are formed by the collective and the individual, and their disciplinary effects. This relates to the idea of the affective economy of care, or, how emotions do things? This includes how emotions are 'transmitted', who creates feels, individual and collective, and whether we can speak of such things as separated, as discrete? As mentioned above, in considering relations of care, we seek to go beyond the idea of transmissions, to examine affective economies as producing and produced; and individuals as not in receipt of, but rather, as active agents in this broader affective economy (albeit 'subject' to countervailing forces and collective efforts). In thinking about the affective economy of suffering and care, we view suffering as assemblages of human bodies, discourses, practices, and as technologies that cannot be allocated exclusively to the singular body of the individual. In terms of the affective dimensions of (collective) suffering and caring, the affective atmosphere, if you will, holds with it the difficulties we face in separating oneself from other people's emotions, and how psychoanalytic dynamics such as enmeshment and dissociation, become part of the relational attempts to 'deal with' suffering. In the following chapters, we articulate these concerns by exploring suffering as individual, interpersonal and collective affect. This become particularly problematic when we explore how seemingly personal suffering is 'dealt with' by formal service providers, within limited understanding of what lies beneath and between these social relations.

Furthermore, we engage with and contribute to queer, feminist and critical race scholarship that emphasizes the importance of engaging with productive possibilities of negative feeling beyond individual psychopathology (Ahmed, 2010; Blackman, 2015; Cvetkovich, 2012; Halberstam, 2011; Love, 2007). Throughout the book, we argue that suffering is and can be a process of becoming. Understanding suffering as being a number of unhappy modes of affect can be both the 'solution to', and site of suffering, concurrently.

Knowing suffering, exploring emotion

Considering suffering, bodies, care and affect from a novel conceptual angle raises concerns about the ontological and epistemological bases of our practices as researchers (Knudsen & Stage, 2015). As Knudsen and Stage (2015) argue, exploring affect challenges many of our practices. How, they ask, do you identify emotions, relations and embodied experiences, when affect is bodily, fleeting and immaterial, not to mention 'in between'? The risk, without challenging our research practices, is to reproduce the very things that we seek to examine and unpack – to explore mere 'bodily suffering' for instance, or the individual experience of physical pain – reifying the separateness of pain and the body, and the emotions that emerge (and converge) therein. Moreover, this book recognises the need to utilise methodologies which produce a sense of presence, relationality and embodiment. The very concepts we seek to explore – concepts such as care, suffering, and distress – necessarily become part of the research process.

In part, we approach this by using different ways into suffering – or what Blackman and Venn call different 'ways of noticing' (Blackman & Venn, 2010). Sometimes this relates to the types of data we have collected. Chapters 3, 4 and 5 utilise a traditional ethnographic methodology, with the research embedded within the scene, the affective atmosphere, and *as participant* in the processes at play. Chapters 1 and 2 utilise more structured qualitative interviews, which provide targeted and snapshot of experiences of narratives of care, suffering and emotions therein. Chapter 6 utilises solicited diaries, written by people living with cancer, which offer another way into the dynamics of suffering, without the (direct) presence of the researcher. In this chapter, we have placed together the interactional/participatory, staged/snapshot and written/narrated to offer different 'ways of noticing' how emotions, affect and care are articulated across difference spheres of suffering. We also examine the different locations from which our accounts/data have been collected – from the institution (hospital setting) to the therapy environment, and to the home and the community setting. Our approach was not to merely gather and focus on literal accounts of suffering, but rather, to explore the discursive components of each site, and how these may 'make up' or could be complicit in suffering and its affective dimensions. As Knudsen and Stage (2015) note, drawing on Haraway, whilst as researchers we shape environments, we are not 'in charge' and thus the world can and does reveal itself in the situations we create. And we acknowledge in the following chapters, that we contribute to the narratives collated, the atmosphere, and the emotions that emerged from our case studies. But these interactions also were beyond our control. These interactions produced the unexpected, and articulated the unruly character of the research-world interface. At times, we intervened, sympathised, offered care and gave recognition to the very accounts which we seek to unpack (the value of care, resilience, the significance of suffering, and impact on relations or discomfort for participating in practice of radical affectivity). In this way, we have been active players in the collective mediation of these stories of suffering, and in the creation of the situated relational ontology of suffering. We are affected by *and* we have affected the research process.

We also offer an interdisciplinary approach, necessarily weaving together the concerns of an anthropologist and a sociologist, as they are articulated in our individual and now collective case studies of suffering. This is an academic assemblage and a relational process in itself. This project has necessarily mutated in directions unanticipated, and has involved tussles between ideas, trajectories and theoretical positions. There is a cultural situatedness to this text which also requires 'outing'. We collected this material in quite different cultural and socioeconomic contexts and this is an important feature of our readings of the emergent data. Chapters 3, 4 and 5 focus on the postcolonial Netherlands, and engage with experiences of suffering across generations in the aftermath of cataclysmic violence and forced migration and suffering caused by everyday racism and marginalisation of the non-white other. Whereas Chapters 1, 2 and 6 focus more on relations of suffering and care (and theoretical and affective dimensions) in the context of settler colonialism in Australia. Biographically, and in terms of research contexts, we also add to the scene as two individuals from economically-richer contexts, with forms of expertise, education and credentials which offer us the opportunity to access these scenes (but also co-create them). Such dynamics are necessarily gendered and imbued with ideas about the 'qualities' of the person, leading us to emphasise that the emergent themes are produced through our relations with our subjects, and their relations with us.

Suffering and (multiple) subjectivities: beyond the individual subject

We argue that suffering needs to be studied in a way that goes beyond an exclusive focus on the human subject. Approaching suffering as an assemblage of human and non-human processes in this way obscures and challenges Cartesian dualism and cautions against a clear demarcation between 'heathy' and 'ill' bodies, carers and the cared for. Our analysis takes as its starting point the idea of 'lived bodies' (Williams & Bendelow, 1998, p. 3). This idea perceives bodies as always in process, emphasising the specificities of material existence while still stressing the importance of cultural and social processes. Such an approach is deeply situated in contemporary body theory, which is 'reintroducing and reformulating bodies as having the capacity to both affect and be affected, with the result that the mind and body are not considered in binary terms' (Blackman, 2008, p. 84). It is important to stress that changes in technology and practices around bodies also challenge our conceptions of the body over time. These changes force us to re-think not only our old ways of understanding bodies, but also our conventional ways of exploring and asking questions about bodies. When the status of the body as 'natural' is contested via transformations in technology, we then must also rethink our paradigms of analysis such as the 'social' and the 'cultural' (Blackman, 2008, p. 3). Following this process, Blackman, in turn, argues that this call to 'think through the body' requires a reshaping of traditional disciplinary boundaries, which separate the physical, biological and social elements of the body to study split between social and natural sciences (ibid.).

The scholarly work that brings the concept of the lived body further began with the ground-breaking study by Dutch anthropologist Annemarie Mol, *The Body Multiple: Ontology in Medical Practice* (2002). In this text, Mol does not focus on the body as a singular entity, but rather argues that the body is an open system that is always connected to other bodies (human and non-human), practices and performances. Mol situates her approach within 'empirical philosophy' based on her empirical work, which involved conducting observations at a hospital in the Netherlands over four years with doctors working on atherosclerosis. Her focus was on studying the practices themselves. Based on this, she argues that there is no one singular medical object but a wide range of practices that produce a multiplicity of objects. Mol argues that, through shifting the focus to practices, 'reality multiplies', and 'what we might think of as a single object may appear to be more than one' (2002, p. vii). In other words, all objects are multiple when considered relative to the practices under which they are the object, because these practices involve different conceptions of reality. Mol takes a social scientific and ethnographic approach to disease, emphasising how understanding the physicality of disease has often been seen as the purview of doctors only, with social scientists adding perspectives on the social meanings of disease. Social scientists have argued that, while doctors attend to the physical aspects of patients, they often overlook the psycho-social elements of 'illness'; that is, living with disease. Mol rejects this perspectival approach, arguing that it loses touch with the physicality of the body, reducing the body to merely something which is interpreted. Mol makes a compelling argument for there being a multiplicity of practices, objects and realities, but does not suggest that this multiplicity results in fragmentation. Rather, Mol engages in an analysis of how various objects 'hang together', arguing that this 'hanging together' is coordinated through contradictions and tensions specific for the situation studied.

Situating our approach within body studies that engage with affect, it is important to state that such engagements characterise the body predominantly in two ways: one the one hand, as open, multiple, and with the capacity to affect and be affected (rather than being closed biological and psychological entities); and, on the other, as always in a process of becoming (Blackman, 2012, p. 2). Following Gregg and Seigworth's (2010) argument that bodies are not stable things or entities, Lisa Blackman (2012, p. 1) cogently argues that 'rather than talk about bodies, we might instead talk of brain-body-world entanglements, and where, how and whether we should attempt to draw boundaries between the human and non-human, self and other, and material and immaterial.' We take Blackman's nexus of 'brain-body-world entanglements' as crucial for our analysis, as it avoids the pitfalls of affect theory scholarship, which perceives affect as only aligned with the non-cognitive, thus perpetuating dichotomies of mind and matter, biology and culture, body and cognition, and physical and psychological. We argue that the theorisation of affect and embodiment requires theories of subject and subjectivity (Blackman, 2012; Navaro-Yashin, 2012).

Outline of this book

Part 1: Suffering, bodies and disease

Chapter 1 undertakes an analysis of how health professionals who are 'caring' for cancer patients (and many who are dying) suffer *in relation*. Drawing on nurses and doctors' accounts of how they process, manage and experience such things as mortality, futility and the end of life, we disrupt notions of care as 'gift' or 'exchange', positioning the professional carer themselves as in, and a part of, suffering. Our aim here is to illustrate how suffering moves across persons in the therapeutic encounter, and that suffering should not be 'treated' as being contained to the patient (who has cancer, or who is nearing death). Rather, suffering circulates, rests on different people, and is supported by particular entrenched social relations and roles. Suffering in this context is in fact an assemblage of roles (professional and lay), desires, expertise, fear, dread and hope – all of which are evident within these difficult and important caring relations. In our focus on the 'labour' of caring for the dying and the character, presence and manifestations of suffering therein, we also explore some of the gendered dimensions of sentimental work, dissociated interpersonal dynamics, and refractory suffering. This chapter places the health professional at centre stage, questioning the nexus between emotions, sentimentality, expertise and professionalism.

Chapter 2 continues the theme of caring-in-relation, and the importance of conceiving suffering as relational. This chapter explores the dynamics of (informal) care for the dying. That is, care offered and provided (or indeed demanded) from families, friends and partners at the end of life. This chapter also explores our theme of suffering-in-relation, and the assemblages of care, but with a focus on exploring the lived experience of caring relations, critiquing the notions of 'carer' and 'cared for', and revealing the day-to-day resistance to normative demands placed on carers at the end of life. In revealing the valorisation of caregiving (as 'natural', 'good', 'rewarding' and 'virtuous'), and how it undermines the lived experience of caring for the dying, we also illustrate how suffering in this context is a collective experience, one that offers a range of moral dilemmas (to 'care', to 'withdraw care', or to 'give us hope') with subsequent affective relations (i.e. shame). The lack of recognition of all those who experience suffering within a particular social context like this both misrepresents the individual (as suffering) and misrecognises the affect and embodied experiences of those who are not acknowledged in this 'scene'.

Part 2: Suffering, the lived body and mobility

Chapter 3 analyses the experiences of intergenerational suffering caused by historical violence, and of family secrecy about the biological relatedness of children fathered by enemy soldiers. In this chapter, we work *with* experiences of historical violence and the practice of secrecy beyond the binary oppositions of conscious and unconscious, intentional and non-intentional, mind and body, health and illness, and culture and psychology. We explore how complex moralities and forms of obligation, and parents' psychological injury incurred during the war, often lead parents to be complicit in the perpetuation of intergenerational suffering. We further argue that the society as a whole is implicit in this complex and contested moral economy of caring. Therefore, we conceptualise suffering as being historically embedded and intergenerationally located. We argue in this chapter that intergenerational suffering must be understood beyond personal psychopathologies, and that we must turn our attention to the fragility of the embodied individual and collective selves.

Chapter 4 analyses the experiences of suffering of transnational adult adoptees caused by everyday racism and marginalisation of the non-white 'other' in contemporary Dutch society. As in Chapter 3, we explore how complex sets of moral obligation to care for children, and in this case, for children that have been perceived as 'abandoned' and 'unwanted' by their biological parents and countries into which they were born, often produces unhappy affect. Our focus in this chapter is an ethnographic exploration of the modalities of the affective politics in which adult adoptees' support group *For Adoptees* engages, in order to inquire into what such engagements allow adoptees to do and become. Our analysis builds on queer, feminist and critical race scholarship that argues for a productive engagement with negative feelings not in terms of pathology (Ahmed, 2010; Blackman, 2015; Cvetkovich, 2012; Halberstam, 2011; Love, 2007), but rather as capable of having creative and productive ends. Furthermore, this chapter explores how therapy cultures – which have commonly been understood as aiming to produce happy affect (e.g. Berlant, 2011; Illouz, 2008; Rose, 1990) – actually mobilise and value negative feelings and employ suffering as a vehicle of ontological transformation.

Part 3: Sites of care, self-help and coping with suffering

Chapter 5 analyses the mobilisation of negative affect by a group healing modality that seeks to heal its subjects' senses of suffering and trauma by intentionally intervening into its participants' pre-cognitive and pre-subjective states. This healing modality that we refer to as a *practice of negative affectivity* mobilises intersubjective exchanges as a way of mutual healing. This poignantly demonstrates the need to think with what Lisa Blackman has termed 'brain-body-world entanglements' (2012, p.1) in arguing that perceiving the rigid boundaries between the human and non-human, self and the other, material and immaterial is counterproductive to our efforts to understand how suffering and radical affectivity can be both the 'solutions to' and sites of suffering. As in Chapter 4, the ethnographic material discussed here urges us to pay attention to therapy cultures that evoke negative affect as a vehicle of ontological transformation. In similar ways to *For Adoptees* gatherings, mutual therapy sessions offer a release of negative affectivity, and a recognition of collective harm and suffering, challenging notions of separateness, and instead offer intense intersubjective encounters that have a focalizing capacity, bringing a sense of 'wholeness'.

In Chapter 6, the emphasis on entanglements moves into the complex sphere of advanced cancer, with a focus on how people living with cancer (terminal/incurable) make sense of the normative, the affective and the embodied. We draw on narratives of living with and dying of cancer to explore the dilemmas of survival (as desired, as normative, as imperative) and the moralities of survival. Drawing on Ahmed (2010) and Berlant (2011), among other scholars, we explore the affective dilemmas in and of cancer survivorship, giving attention to how other, often less obvious things, induce suffering (rather than merely disease). This involves a critique of normative expectations, collective demands and clinical knowing – introducing these and other dynamics as complicit in suffering. Here, we again seek to emphasise that suffering does not emerge from disease, lie in the person, or is an inevitability – rather, it is the creative outcome of a complex assemblage of human and non-human actors, and must be viewed as such if we are to support all those who experience it.

In the Conclusion, we review what has been explored in the book, outlining the key conceptual ideas and offering a sense of where these concepts may lead in the future. This includes the importance and significance of the affective assemblage, the notion of suffering-in-relation, and what specific areas may be the subjects of future research.

Notes

1 See also Ahmed (2004, 2010).
2 Most anthropological studies have focused on studying emotions from a cultural-relativist and cross-cultural perspective. In the 1980s and 1990s, anthropologists engaged in an effort to demonstrate how emotions are culturally constructed, positioning non-Western cultures in opposition to the West, which was understood to treat emotions as psychological and biological. Aiming to destabilize the Eurocentric notion of the 'self', this scholarship focused on expressions of emotions as determined by culture and language. Such scholarship, like much of the anthropological work at the time, focused primarily on the human as a sole producer of emotions, through language and discourse (e.g. Lutz, 1988, Lutz and Abu-Lughod, 1990). For a more recent, notable exception, see Navaro-Yashin (2012).

References

Ahmed, S. (2004a). Affective economies. *Social Text*, 79(22), pp. 117–139.

Ahmed, S. (2004b). *The Cultural Politics of Emotion*. New York: Routledge.

Ahmed, S. (2010). *The Promise of Happiness*. Durham, NC: Duke University Press.

Ahmed, S. (2014). *Willful Subjects*. Durham, NC and London: Duke University Press.

Bauman, Z. (2013). *Liquid Modernity*. John Wiley.

Berlant, L. G. (2011). *Cruel Optimism*. Durham, NC: Duke University Press.

Blackman, L. (2008). *The Body: The Key Concepts*. Oxford, New York: Berg.

Blackman, L. (2012). *Immaterial Bodies: Affect, Embodiment, Mediation*. Thousand Oaks, CA: Sage.

Blackman, L. (2015). Affective politics, debility and hearing voices: towards a feminist politics of ordinary suffering. *Feminist Review*, 111(4), pp. 25–41.

Blackman, L. & Venn, C. (2010). 'Affect'. *Body & Society*, 16(1), pp. 1–6.

Bourdieu, P. (1999). *The Weight of the World: Social Suffering in Contemporary Society*. UK: Alhoda.

Bracke, P., Christiaens, W. & Wauterickx, N. (2008). The pivotal role of women in informal care. *Journal of Family Issues*, 29(10), pp. 1348–1378.

Braidotti, R. (2013). *Posthuman*. Cambridge, UK, Malden, MA: Polity Press.

Brennan, T. (2004). *The Transmission of Affect*. New York, London: Cornell University Press.

Bubeck, D. (1995). *Care, Gender, and Justice*. Oxford: Clarendon Press.

Clement, G. (1996). *Care, Autonomy, and Justice*. Boulder, CO: Westview Press.

Clough, P. (2004). Future matters: Technoscience, global politics, and cultural criticism. *Social Text*, 22(3), pp. 1–23.

Clough, P. T. (2007). Introduction. In Clough, P. T. & Halley, J. eds, *The Affective Turn: Theorizing the Social*. Durham, NC: Duke University Press, pp. 1–34.

Cohen, S. (2013). *States of Denial: Knowing About Atrocities and Suffering*. John Wiley & Sons.

Coole, D. & Frost, S. (2010). *New Materialisms: Ontology, Agency, and Politics*. Durham, NC: Duke University Press.

Csordas, T., ed. (1994). *Embodiment and Experience: The Existential Ground of Culture and Self*. Cambridge: Cambridge University Press.

Cvetkovich, A. (2012). *Depression: A Public Feeling*. Durham, NC: Duke University Press.

Das, V., Kleinman, A., Ramphele, M. & Reynolds, P. (2000) Berkeley, CA, London: University of California Press.

Davies, W. (2014). *The limits of neoliberalism: Authority, sovereignty and the logic of competition*. London; Thousand Oaks, CA: Sage.

Deleuze, G. & Guattari, F. (1986). *Kafka: Toward a Minor Literature*. Minneapolis, MN: University of Minnesota Press.

Deleuze, G. & Guattari, F. (1987). *A Thousand Plateaus: Capitalism and Schizophrenia*. Minneapolis, MN: University of Minnesota Press.

Diedrich, L. (2015). Illness as assemblage: The case of hystero-epilepsy. *Body & Society*, 21, pp. 66–90.

Dragojlovic, A. (2015). Affective geographies: Intergenerational hauntings, bodily affectivity and multiracial subjectivities. *Subjectivity*, 8, pp. 315–334.

Farmer, P. (1996). On suffering and structural violence: A view from below. *Daedalus*, pp. 261–283.

Finch, J. & Groves, D., eds. (1983). *A Labour of Love*. London: Routledge.

Fisher, B. & Tronto, J. (1990). Toward a feminist theory of care. In Abel, E. and Nelson, M., eds., *Circles of Care*. Albany, NY: State University of New York Press, pp. 35–62.

Gilligan, C. (1982). *In a Different Voice*. Cambridge, MA: Harvard University Press.

Goodin, R. (1985). *Protecting the Vulnerable*. Chicago: University of Chicago Press.

Gordon, S. et al. (1996). *Caregiving*. Philadelphia, PA: University of Pennsylvania Press.

Graham, H. (1991). The concept of caring in feminist research. *Sociology*, 25(1), pp. 61–78.

Halberstam, J. J. (2011). *The Queer Art of Failure*. Durham, NC: Duke University Press.

Harvey, D. (2005). *Spaces of Neoliberalization: Towards a Theory of Uneven Geographical Development* (Vol. 8). Franz Steiner Verlag.

Held, V., ed. (1995). *Justice and Care*. Boulder, CO: Westview Press.

Held, V. (2005). *The Ethics of Care*. Oxford: Oxford University Press.

Illouz, E. (2008). *Saving the Modern Soul: Therapy, Emotions, and the Culture of Self-help*. Berkeley, CA: University of California Press.

Kittay, E. (1999). *Love's Labor*. New York: Routledge.

Kittay, E. & Feder, E. (2002). *The Subject of Care*. Lanham, MD: Rowman and Littlefield Publishers.

Kleinman, A. (1988). *The Illness Narratives: Suffering, Healing, and the Human Condition*. New York: Basic Books.

Kleinman, A. (1992). Local worlds of suffering: An interpersonal focus for ethnographies of illness experience. *Qualitative Health Research*, 2(2), pp. 127–134.

Kleinman, A. (1997). Everything that really matters. *Harvard Theological Review*, 90(3), pp. 315–335.

Kleinman, A., Das, V. & Lock, M. M. (1997). *Social Suffering*. Berkeley, CA: University of California Press.

Knudsen, B. T. & Stage, C. (2015). Introduction: Affective methodologies. In Knudsen, B. T. & Stage, C., eds, *Affective Methodologies*. Basingstoke: Palgrave Macmillan UK, pp. 1–22.

Larrabee, M. J. (1993). *An Ethic of Care*. Hove: Psychology Press.

Latimer, J. (2008). Introduction: Body, knowledge, worlds. *The Sociological Review*, 56(s2), pp. 1–22.

Leys, R. (2011a). The turn to affect: A critique. *Critical Inquiry*, 37(3), pp. 434–472.

Leys, R. (2011b). Affect and intention: A reply to William E. Connolly. *Critical Inquiry*, 37(3), pp. 799–805.

Love, H. (2007). *Feeling Backward: Loss and the Politics of Queer History*. Cambridge, MA: Harvard University Press.

Lutz, C. (1988). *Unnatural Emotions: Everyday Sentiments on A Micronesian Atoll and Their Challenge to Western Theory*. Chicago: University of Chicago Press.

Lutz, C. A. & Abu-Lughod, L., eds. (1990). *Language and the Politics of Emotion*. Cambridge: Cambridge University Press.

Marecek, J. (2006). Social suffering, gender, and women's depression. In C. L. M. Keyes, ed., *Women and Depression: A Handbook for the Social, Behavioral, and Biomedical Sciences*. New York: Cambridge University Press, pp. 283–308.

Massumi, B. (2002). *Parables for the Virtual: Movement, Affect, Sensation*. Durham, NC: Duke University Press.

Mol, A. (2002). *The Body Multiple: Ontology in Medical Practice*. Durham, NC: Duke University Press.

Mol, A. (2008). *The Logic of Care*. Abingdon, Oxon: Routledge.

Munro, R. & Belova, O. (2008). The body in time: Knowing bodies and the 'interruption' of narrative. *The Sociological Review*, 56(s2), 85–99.

Navaro-Yashin, Y. (2012). *The Make-Believe Space: Affective Geography in a Postwar Polity*. Durham, NC: Duke University Press.

Parker G., (1993). *With This Body*. Buckingham: Open University Press.

Poole, M. & Isaacs, D. (1997). Caring: A gendered concept. *Women's Studies International Forum*, 20(4), pp. 529–536.

Rose, N. (1990). *Governing the Soul: The Shaping of the Private Self*. London & New York: Routledge.

Rousseau, J. J. (1920). *The Social Contract: & Discourses* (No. 660). London: J M Dent.

Sayer, A. (2005). Class, moral worth and recognition. *Sociology*, 39(5), pp. 947–963.

Seigworth, G. J. & Gregg, M. (2010). An inventory of shimmers. In Gregg, M. & Seigworth, G. J., eds, *The Affect Theory Reader*. Durham, NC: Duke University Press, pp. 1–27.

Shildrick, M. & Steinberg, D. L. (2015). Estranged bodies: Shifting paradigms and the biomedical imaginary. *Body & Society*, 21, pp. 3–19.

Shilling, C. (2003). *The Body and Social Theory*. London: Sage Publications.

Springer, S. & Honours, B. A. (2016). *The Discourse of Neoliberalism: An Anatomy of a Powerful Idea*. London: Rowman & Littlefield International.

Thrift, N. (2008). *Non-Representational Theory: Space, Politics, Affect*. New York: Routledge.

Tronto, J. (1998). An ethic of care. *Generations*, 22(3), pp. 15–20.

Tronto, J., (1993). *Moral Boundaries*. New York: Routledge.

Twigg, J. & Atkin, K. (1994). *Carers Perceived*. Buckingham: Open University Press.

Ungerson, C. (1983). Why do women care? In Finch, J. & Groves, D., eds, *A Labour of Love: Women, Work and Caring*. London: Routledge & Kegan Paul, pp. 31–49.

Ungerson, C. (1987). *Policy is Personal*. New York: Tavistock.

West, R. (2002). The right to care. In Kittay, E. F. & Feder, E., eds, *The Subject of Care*. Lanham, MD: Rowman & Littlefield.

Wetherell, M. (2012). *Affect and Emotion: A New Social Science Understanding*. Los Angeles: Sage Publications.

Williams, F. (2001). In and beyond New Labour: towards a new political ethics of care. *Critical social policy*, 21(4), 467–493.

Williams, S. J. & Bendelow, G. (1998). *The Lived Body: Sociological Themes, Embodied Issues*. London and New York, Routledge.

Wise, J. M. (2005). Assemblage. In Stivale, C. J., ed., *Gilles Deleuze: Key Concepts*. Chesham: Acumen, pp. 77–87.

Part 1

Suffering, bodies and disease

1 Who's suffering?

Professional care and private suffering

Introduction

As we outlined in the Introduction, suffering presents as an affective assemblage, of which relations of care (both formal and informal) are an inextricable part. Suffering is necessarily *about* care and in this way, it is also necessarily about others, and about the intersubjective realm. This includes consideration of what caring (or non-caring) relations may or may not offer to 'us' (carer) and 'them' (patient/ person). And crucially, for this chapter, it raises questions of where suffering is, or lies, in the context of caring relations. In the context of affliction or even the dying process, suffering has generally been explored simply *through* the experience of the person who is ill. Or, in the context of work on bereavement, through the experience of loved ones, carers or families who are themselves suffering. The 'caring' professions, as it were, including nurses and doctors, who are tasked with 'treating' and ameliorating suffering, have not figured in these explorations to any meaningful extent. This is an artefact of the tendency to construct the carer/care for dichotomy within the context of the institutionalisation and professionalisation of care in modernity. But what do those working in the 'caring' professions experience, and what is their contribution to the inter-subjectivity of suffering? Are they merely distanced, dispassionate, 'professionals' and *being supportive*? Or is there much more to, and underlying, (formal) caring encounters than the carer and the sufferer duality? Where does suffering really lie within this caring assemblage? What does suffering do, exactly?

The suffering of doctors and nurses, we posit here, reflects enduring problematic divisions and erroneous distinctions within the formal caring dynamic (e.g. cared for, caring; *in* pain, *treating* pain; see Chattoo & Ahmad, 2008). We seek to challenge and unravel the (in this case formal) affective relations of care, and the moral, ethical and affective struggles that *being in* and *being with* suffering may induce. We ask, where does suffering really lie in this encounter? Who is holding it, sharing in it, and acting *in relation* to it? To answer these questions, we offer an analysis that pursues a relational ontology of *being in* care (rather than offering or receiving it), and how feelings move across persons to create particular atmospheres (i.e. dread, hope, hopelessness). In this way we aim to explore care as the relational context of – and for – suffering. Of particular importance here is how the silence of clinicians (as feeling) has reified such exchange models (carer/cared for), and dualisms of care as being 'provided' and 'received'. This, in turn, locates suffering erroneously within the realm of the 'cared for'; an assumption that is not only inaccurate, but potentially undermines the care provided and viability of caring practices.

We focus on a particularly challenging site of caring relations and affective exchange – those at the end of life – to explore how *being with* suffering is in fact *being in* suffering for healthcare professionals. That is, we aim to 'out' the feelings of clinicians in order to illustrate the circulation of affect within healthcare professionals' own relations of care, and the co-production of suffering as an affective assemblage. As Sara Ahmed argues, affective dynamics have generative qualities: 'We are moved by things. In being moved we make things' (2010, p. 25). This is in turn the case in medicine, and that it does indeed produce 'things'.

In this chapter, we draw on a particular field of medicine and nursing to explore the inherent relationality and inter-subjective character of suffering during *and* in care. We examine the particular context of medical futility and the (challenging) transition to the end of life. This is a challenging relational moment in the therapeutic landscape, unsettling the (multifaceted) desires of its subjects (e.g. doctor–longevity/core; patient–hope/recovery), and thus offers a prominent site of interpersonal tension, tussle and often suffering (MacArtney et al., 2015, 2017). This moment also challenges all actors in the assemblage of care, including doctors, nurses, families, and the person who is dying. As we will show in the narratives offered below, in the context of negotiating treatment and care in oncology, palliative, and end-of-life settings, doctors and nurses themselves engage in what is often known as 'sentimental work'. This work involves intense interpersonal relations, and it raises questions around *who* is suffering, for what reasons, and to what end (i.e. survival, longevity, denial). Thus, this chapter will focus on the 'labour of caring' for the dying, and the character and underpinnings of suffering therein for doctors and nurses in particular.

We argue that while the person who is dying is rightly recognised as an important 'suffering subject', there are other individuals and affective dimensions that have been often unappreciated in this moment. These include subjects who cannot be separated from the experience of the person who is dying and their suffering. The affective atmosphere, in the context of advanced cancer, futility and the end of life, holds (and is held up by) many actors in the life (and death) of the individual person. These actors include doctors and nurses, who, in seeking to professionally 'manage' suffering, suffer themselves, experiencing enmeshment, melancholia, dissociation, and many other conditions in their relational attempts to 'deal with' the suffering of an Other. We will use this moment to illustrate how suffering is a collective act, as well part of an individual narrative/experience. We interrogate this by asking: what lies beneath the surface of therapeutic social relations and professional acts and performances?

In exploring suffering as a relational assemblage, this chapter places the clinician (whether doctor or nurse) at centre stage in suffering as well as the 'delivery' of care. This aim augments Chapter 2, which focuses on suffering amongst informal carers (family members and partners) for people who are dying; and Chapter 6, which focuses on the experiences of people living with advanced cancer. In the current chapter, we emphasise the importance of an understanding that suffering ripples across institutional, interprofessional, and interpersonal social relations. Moreover, we emphasise that clinical/psycho-social notions are often used to make sense of the affective dimensions of care for health professionals who evade the relational dynamics of care and collective suffering. The 'good professional' is often conflated with the distanced, yet compassionate, provider of care (Broom et al., 2016).

A good example of the reductive conception of care and suffering, regularly used in the therapeutic literature is 'compassion fatigue' (e.g. Abendroth & Flannery, 2006). This concept aims to normalise a withdrawal from 'feeling things' on the part of health professionals. The concept of 'compassion fatigue' does little to account for the *affective entanglements* of professional (medical and nursing) work. Nor does it account for the intensities circulating between bodies (Dragojlovic, 2015; and see also the Introduction to this book). In fact, such notions reinforce spurious assumptions that suffering lies with the patient (in this case, the patient who is dying), and that a unilateral professional compassion (which waxes and wanes) operates in relation to a non-specific Other (who holds and experiences *the* suffering). In unsettling this persistent representation, we focus here on how suffering, and the affective dimensions therein, lie across persons at the end of life.

We also posit here that it is more than merely clinicians being part of suffering; rather, they offer things to these social relations including: a sense of their own failure to help or master disease; their anticipatory grief of a loss of therapeutic alliance; and, an anticipated loss of personal relationships with patients. These affective dimensions are often encoded in the rationalities of the therapeutic encounter, and (we argue) produce forms of suffering. These forms include the need to 'hold on' to life even in the 'face of death'; and a collusion between doctor and patient that articulates the frustrations across persons (doctor, patient, family) (McNamara et al., 1995; Melvin & Oldham, 2009; Zimmermann, 2012). For these reasons, and others outlined below, we posit the urgent need for clinicians to become viewed as part of, and experiencing suffering; that this should be articulated and conceptualised in relational terms, and in turn be seen as produced by the micro (i.e. relationship loss, anticipated disconnection) and the macro (i.e. the ambitions of professionals and the failure of professional projects for life prolongment).

Suffering as a therapeutic and inter-subjective relation

The problematic 'treatment' of suffering within the therapeutic encounter has emerged from a complex history of the clinical milieu separating 'professions' from their (and others') emotions. It makes sense that the language of much clinical training and practice guidelines, whether in medicine or nursing, is based primarily on the amelioration of the suffering of a *dying other*. Work in palliative and end-of-life care has explicitly or implicitly articulated suffering in relation to the person who is dying rather than the collective potential experience or role of the clinician in perpetuating or creating suffering (Denier et al., 2010; Mol, 2008; Morita et al., 2004). The premise of the hospice movement was to better address the 'total pain' of *the individual* who was dying, in all its complex intermingling facets, including the physiological, spiritual, social, relational and psychological (Broom, 2015; Morris & Thomas, 2007). The clinical literature has thus tended to portray suffering as being located within a singular person rather than dispersed across persons (those paid and unpaid, those sick, dying, bereaved or 'well') (e.g. Back et al., 2009; Denier et al., 2010; Friedrichsen & Strang, 2003; McSteen & Peden-McAlpine, 2006). The assumption here is that understanding and 'managing' suffering should necessarily be directed at the patient and their family/carers. This assumption, we posit, is erroneous, and may also be (at least partially) responsible for suffering itself.

Presuming that suffering lies securely with the ill or dying person, or with their carer, and is strictly about 'the threat of imminent death' results in the concealment of important interpersonal 'exchanges' including transference, countertransference, and projection (Broom & Kirby, 2013; MacArtney et al., 2015a, b). The classic psychoanalytic dynamics of enmeshment and dissociation thus become part of the relational attempts to 'deal with' suffering that actually produce suffering. The multiple facets of suffering at the end of life, however we name them – whether 'loss', 'grief', 'hopelessness', 'care', 'compassion', 'hope', 'sense of failure' – are each dependent on a set of social ties, and relational experiences, and are necessarily about the potential for these to be disrupted or broken (in the context of dying). There has been little consideration of what the professional's 'sentimentality' and (often implicit) suffering may contribute or offer to the dynamic. Here, we posit that suffering is experienced, embodied and co-produced by health professionals, who are themselves struggling with the challenges of the limits of human life, and the limits of their professional projects. This is differentiated according to the values of different professional groups (both self-imposed and externally ascribed) and the extent to which they are allowed, and able to, express forms of suffering emergent both from these perceived limitations of their role/capabilities.

Current logics of practice and care: 'denial', 'compassion fatigue', 'burnout'

There is no shortage of available psycho-social concepts seeking to capture forms of professional and lay affect in the context of futility, death and dying. Whether referred to in terms of patient 'denial' or 'anticipatory grief', or (for professionals) in terms of 'compassion fatigue', or 'professional burnout', there is an affective industry of sorts reifying the binary understanding of suffering (Kellehear, 1984). What these concepts have in common is they emphasise suffering as located within the person – not across persons. *Anticipatory grief*, for example, captures the anticipated loss of the person who is dying, whether from the perspective of the person themselves, or the significant other (in the future), again locating suffering firmly as about the individual's death (Cheng et al., 2013; Nielsen et al., 2016; Sweeting & Gilhooly, 1990). *Compassion fatigue* refers to the supposedly diminishing returns of compassion in highly emotional contexts, of which hospice care is a good example (Abendroth & Flannery, 2006; Slocum-Gori et al., 2013). Health professionals faced with continual patient pain and suffering, develop various affective dispositions including hopelessness, lack of compassion or capacity to 'properly care' (Ablett & Jones, 2007; Adamle & Ludwick, 2005; Graham, 2006). Often linked with *professional burnout* (see Broom, 2015), compassion fatigue reflects a psycho-social framing of why (some) professionals seem to care less over time and as they are exposed to others' suffering (Potter et al., 2010; Sprang et al., 2007). This firmly positions suffering as located with the dying Other (that is, the patient) rather than acknowledging the forms of relational suffering that the clinician might be experiencing.

Such concepts, and others in the palliative care literature, are based on an assumption that the ultimate source of suffering lies in the total pain of the person dying (e.g. Boston et al., 2011). This fundamentally misrepresents what and how professionals *experience* and *contribute* to suffering. In fact, suffering moves across persons, is multifactorial, embedded in inter-personal and professional ambitions, and is the product of a series of contradictory expectations for formal care/rs (technical skills versus human caring behaviours). Health professionals, we posit, are in fact active participants in the co-production of suffering as an affective assemblage. A doctors' experience of grief and sadness at failing to provide hope or cure, meaningfully and potently contribute to the experience of illness and the dying process (for the patient and their family). Thus, suffering circulates across this social environment, with this experience being produced, often subtly, in and by relations (and with its contributors often concealed by the pursuit of 'professionalism' and 'distance').

In seeking to reconsider conceptions of suffering as relational, we focus here on what professionals feel and contribute, taking into account their personal experiences and professional ambitions. In doing this, we need to consider what professional care actually constitutes; is it merely a commercial transaction, gift, duty, or all of these? What is the perceived responsibility of the professional, and how does this flow through to the forms of suffering that ensue? What is the character of the perceived or technical contract between professional and patient (consider here ideas espoused by the Hippocratic oath for medicine, or the work of Florence Nightingale and others in nursing)? How might the suffering of the professional flow through to the suffering of the person who is dying? To *not intimately care*, as we will explore below, is viewed as the key to survival in the palliative and hospice care setting, and personal suffering on the part of the professional remains something of a taboo (Broom et al., 2013, 2014). This sits in contrast to the persistent interpersonal caring relationship, and the components therein of gift or sacrifice. The question of who exactly is suffering, and for what reasons, is what we seek to raise here, with professionals not merely offering a gift of care (and suffering as a result) but actively grieving a range of things including: the contradictions/limitations of their professional projects and skills; their horror of their own (and collective) mortality; the injustice of illness and treatment outcomes; and, the sense of interpersonal failure that accompanies dying.

Notes on fieldwork

Below, we draw on interviews with doctors and nurses conducted by Alex Broom in 2011, 2012 and 2013 (20 doctors and 20 nurses, all working in Queensland, Australia) in a range of oncological and palliative care specialties. Participants were either involved in the referral of patients to palliative and/or end-of-life care, or in the caring for people who had already been referred. This resulted in over 40 interviews oriented toward the art of delivering a terminal prognosis, and the dynamics of supporting people to shift to, or receive palliative care. Each clinician was required to initiate discussions about futility, the lack of any meaningful curative interventions remaining, and, ultimately, the dying process. These moments require, or necessarily involve, intensive emotional 'work' from patients, carers and professionals. Often, as we show, there is a division of 'emotional work' between doctors and nurses. Suffering, as it emerges, lies not with just the person who is dying, but at the inter-subjective and relational levels of all involved with the process.

Emotions at work

In line with what is outlined above, the interviews focused on exploring how these Australian-based doctors and nurses managed affective dimensions of 'letting go', caring and their own emotions (if acknowledged) in the context of medical futility and the transition to the end of life. Often this discussion centred on tensions between the *act of professional work* vis-à-vis participation in *humanistic* relations of care. Such priorities were frequently viewed as contradictory and producing competing logics of practice. Specifically, healthcare professionalisation has seen the routinisation and systematisation of medical work (Bailey et al., 2011; Graham, 2006; Gray, 2010; Miller et al., 2008; Nettleton et al., 2008). This has been partial, and as we posit here, often functions to conceal the persistent and challenging affective dimensions of care. Moreover, what transformations in health work (including those related to neoliberalism) *do* to affective relations of care. An emphasis on the emotional challenges clinicians face – including dilemmas around the affective atmosphere at work – we argue, helps us make sense of broader dynamics including those of 'over-treatment', collusion between doctor, nurse and patients, 'denying futility' and collective 'resistance to palliative care' (Broom et al., 2014; Broom et al., 2016; MacArtney et al., 2016). These dynamics can be meaningfully understood as (partially) produced by clinicians' experiences of suffering-in-relation. Below, we unpack these considerations regarding such things as: doctors' emotional responses to 'walking people to their grave' and the subsequent dynamics of detachment and dissociation as well as the attempts of nurses to '[get] close enough but not too close' in their relations with patients.

Doctors' emotions when 'walking people to their grave'

The interviews with the doctors tended to focus on how they articulated the affective dimensions of their therapeutic relationships, with particular reference to conversations about futility, dying, and the transition to the end of life. What did they feel? What did they do if it was difficult, and what was the impact on conversations, decisions and relationships? These were not easy conversations to have with doctors as the 'subjects' of research. They often wanted to convey opinions or rational responses to questions such as 'is this difficult for you and in what ways?', 'what do you do with the emotional intensity of telling people they are dying?', or 'does it get to you and how do you deal with it?' However, with the development of rapport in the interviews, with gradual movement toward the topic of how *they feel*, for many it was possible to access the affective dimensions of their work – or, at least how they represented it. As we shall show below, the doctors interviewed often had ongoing, very personal struggles, *and suffered*, in response to their patients' mortality. This relational suffering in the therapeutic encounter is perhaps unsurprising, but has received very little attention from the social sciences. This reflects a broader neglect of emotions in medical sociology (Bendelow & Williams, 1998; Graham, 2006; Nettleton et al., 2008). 'Telling them they will die' was not just professionally difficult or fatiguing, but rather, it was a powerful site of suffering for many of the interviewees themselves and was talked about as 'physically hurting' the clinician. More than a matter of professional care, the oncologists often felt this hurt in their bodies, and often talked about suffering together (often in silence) with their patient, as well as with their patient's family. In this way, it is not 'managing pain' of an Other, but also experiencing pain and suffering, and this has effects, and impacts upon, the therapeutic relationship (this will be discussed at greater length below).

For example, David claimed that he was able to tolerate those who had 'had a good life',[1] but for those 'young ones' or ones that 'bring in prams', his response was highly emotional (even if this was not transparent in the therapeutic encounter):

David: The very young ones, I've had 30-year-olds, or 27-year-olds die. They usually hang out until the last [minute], I would say you know, almost until the last month or so, they just don't want to be handed over to the palliative care team. And it's not only them, it's their families . . . it's still heartbreaking to have to tell them, with the mother or father in the room, that there is just nothing more I can offer them . . . It's really hard to walk people up to their grave and say 'okay, jump in'. And that's what they think, [oncologists] feel their position is when they have to say 'stop now'. . . . The ones that I really struggle with, are the ones that have young kids. And I've seen the kids a lot. Because, you know the thing is, a lot of young parents have nowhere to put their babies, and they'll come to clinic with their prams. That's just, I mean that kind of thing, you actually dread it, a few months before it's actually going to happen . . . [Physician, Female]

Angus reflects that his emotional response to particular patients (and their families) can be influenced by the life stories of those patients:

Angus: . . . you do think, 'okay, he's [sic] about my age,' or 'he's got kids around my age', you know. I've got a number of young women, who had bad disease, and they've got little kids, and you feel for them, you really feel for them. Sometimes you'll just have one of those bad days where I come out of here thinking 'oh Christ, how many people have I told they're going to die today?' [Surgery, Male]

The presence of children was often raised as the most difficult emotional dynamic of the therapeutic encounter, yet, these doctors' emotional difficulties, and forms of relational suffering therein, extended well beyond the 'dying mothers with children' scenario. Their own struggles with the emotions of futility, mortality and the strength of their professional and personal desire to offer to extend life (often regardless of the impact on quality of life) meant that across their encounters, and particularly at the point of futility, their own interpersonal struggles were magnified. The affective atmosphere, of which they are both holding up, and held by, shapes the offerings of particular clinical pathways (i.e. offer further options, continue active treatment, resist referral to palliative care). This – and an underlying grief of what may be to come – was often acknowledged in the interviews, and was driven at least in part by the doctor's own emotional state, despite being represented as scientific, objective or evidence-based (Melvin & Oldham, 2009; Temel et al., 2010). This was explained in various ways, and as we see below in Arnold's interview, often as a practice of protecting the patient from difficult emotions.

Arnold describes 'knowing in your heart' that the situation is hopeless, but 'offering things' to bolster their hopes and mood. This bypasses the emotions of the doctor, and pushes them onto the patient and oncological action as protective of the patient:

Arnold: So often times if patients get a recurrence it's a situation where you sort of know in your heart that they're likely to succumb [to] their disease. But often we sort of convince ourselves that we can, you know, fix it . . . Yeah, and when you're dealing with those patients, you sort of try and be positive, even though you know, if it comes back, you sort of know that it's not looking too good for them, yeah. [Surgeon, Male]

Part of the problem with the rationalisation that it is 'patient feelings' being looked after rather than oncologists' own desires and feelings. The oncologists' own affective contributions to the trajectory of care are concealed.

And in effect, much rationalisation of 'trying other things' may in fact be embedded in the suffering of doctors at the prospect not being 'able to fix them' or 'giving up' on the patient. There is some psychosocial research on this and the notions of *collusion* or *mutual pretence*, as examples, are regularly discussed within the clinical literature (mostly in relation to palliative care, rather than in oncology contexts) (Smith et al., 2012; The et al., 2000; Zimmermann, 2007). These notions capture the dynamic of 'collective denial' or strategic silences in therapeutic encounters, but neither really acknowledges the emotions, vulnerabilities and forms of suffering experienced by doctors. This lack of acknowledgment, in turn, contributes to the reification of the medical 'expert' as (largely) dispassionate, objective, scientific and rational. The patient and/or their family are positioned here as being vulnerable, emotional, susceptible, irrational, or lacking in perspective. One can see that this erroneous misrepresentation of actors – in terms of the affective dimensions of care – has considerable implications for the character of care provided over the course of (in this case) cancer treatment and the timing of discussions about futility and palliative and end-of-life care. Yet, this was often rationalised as being 'all about patients' and not actually embedded in the feelings of the doctors themselves:

Jeffrey: [We will say to patients] . . . 'we've got something for you!' We go, 'here's a trial, you could go on this?' And they [the patient] go, 'well, this must be good you know, if it's a trial it's something fantastic.' Even though you could go to great lengths to say, 'this is not going to cure your lung cancer' . . . people [patients] often have unrealistic expectations. [Medical Oncology, Male]

In Jeffrey's short quote, and in many of the other participants' narratives, one can see concurrently the *explicit acknowledgement* of the role of emotions in shaping what is offered to their cancer patients, yet a *clear dismissiveness* of their own emotions in the trajectory of care (i.e. the problem is patients' 'unrealistic expectations'). 'Holding on', 'offering more' and embarking on treatments with 'diminishing returns' were positioned by the doctors as 'what patients want' rather than an articulation of the doctor's affective contributions. As discussion within the interviews continued, and as we see in Diane's narrative below, it emerged that the oncologists are also protecting themselves through strategies of denying emotions, with a backstage reality of private suffering:

Diane: So there are a lot of oncologists who just don't have that art, of being able [to communicate dying] . . . I think that's just protecting themselves, maybe?
Interviewer: From what?
Diane: Well, from the emotions! It's not easy! Like you can't, you know, you can't go home after having told maybe three people that they have nothing left, you can't go home normal that day, it does affect you, and then you just, you know, you're quite low for, for, well for at least the rest of the evening, and the night until the next morning. It has to affect you, because we're all just human beings, right? You can't be numb to it. [Physician, Female]

The above reflection was in fact quite unusual within this group of oncologists. The reflection touched on a rarely described 'back stage' reality that was clearly present in some form for all of the participants – there were forms of suffering that did or *should not* appear in the workplace, were not accommodated in understandings of influences on decisions or treatment trajectories, and were not discussed between health professionals (see also Broom et al., 2016). Moreover, their own emotional struggles were regularly projected onto patients (e.g. 'they have unrealistic expectations'), with their own feelings of failure, grief or (anticipatory) loss covered up by a subject position that disallowed these very affective dimensions (cf. Back et al., 2009; Brown et al., 2009). The solution, as it were, was to implement various strategies to minimise the acknowledgement of emotions and suffering therein, within relations of care.

Doctors, detachment, suffering

It was interesting to consider what dynamics would emerge when emotions were considered just too difficult to acknowledge, process, or even incorporate within oncological work. While oncologists have regularly been pushed to engage more with the person (rather than disease) in their interactions with patients (Fox, 2006; Fox & Lief, 1963), it is worth considering the extent to which tendencies within professional work actually reflect a response to the threat, and reality of, emotional burden or forms of suffering amongst medical professionals, and for oncologists in particular. Various problematic notions, including that of 'detached concern' (Fox, 2006; Fox & Lief, 1963) have emerged, reflecting a dis-ease with emotions more broadly in medicine. This is reflected in some of the interviewees' narratives where they discuss strategies of detachment, withdrawal or even dissociation. Holding 'quick consultations' which *could not* accommodate emotional issues was one strategy described in the interviews, often, as we shall see below, shifting the emotional burden (and dialogue) of the therapeutic trajectory to nurses:

Michael: Unfortunately, I've got patients queuing up at the door. I've got to see 25 patients today, and [emotional engagement] is just not possible. So I often, the shortcut is to, particularly with those who have got unresolved emotional issues, is to divert that to some colleagues, so either nursing or social work colleagues. [Medical Oncology, Male]

Michael's response provided one strategy of diversion, whereas Oscar, Alan and Craig each viewed 'actually caring' in therapeutic relationships as impossible and the practice of 'taking emotion out of it' the only way to operate:

Oscar: I don't find it [referral to palliative care] hard. It's not that there's no emotion attached to it, there isn't a lot of emotion attached to it, you do what you can, and then move on to the next person . . . with respect, because the people [doctors] who really care, don't last, because it's too you know, to actually carry that emotional baggage with you, you're not going to sustain yourself . . . [Medical Oncology, Male]

Alan: . . . you get into a model of pragmatism about pointing out what is and is not possible for them. Um, relating empathically with them about that, and sometimes those are difficult conversations, sometimes they last longer than you would like . . . [Urology, Male]

Craig: . . . I do take the emotion out of it, and it's very factual. I don't know if that's offensive to people, but that's just the way I do it . . . if you get overly involved emotionally, you're not going to give necessarily the best care, because your inside, or your decision-making process is blurred. So, you can still feel for people, but at the end of the day, yeah you're not overly involved emotionally . . . I stopped going to funerals a long time ago . . . [Haematology, Male]

These quotes suggest how the need to reduce emotional expression, and side-line the affective dimensions of formalised caring relations, is put into practice by some of these doctors. Reducing exposure to the 'realities' of human mortality and distress (i.e. funerals), and cutting down the time spent in medical consultations which involve discussion of futility and the dying process, were just some of the ways of ensuring that one does not 'care too much'. Of course, such strategies concealed – and often not very effectively – participants' rather torn relationship with their own emotions and suffering. However, not all participants saw emotion reduction as the core to survival within the profession, with a minority viewing the recognition of emotions as part of the value of this form of work:

Samuel: I mean, emotionally it can be difficult, and the point of view that I'm cutting myself off . . . well, I think that's a bit of a cop out. And in fact, the point in time when I do that, is going to be the time when you're really missing out on something. Because even though it might be emotionally draining, if you just stand back and say, 'well, here you go, on your way,' that's a problem, I think, well, you might say that you're protecting yourself, but in fact you're missing out on some [thing] . . . that's not a very healthy approach, not to get involved. [Medical Oncology, Male]

There is nuance in their approaches to, and views on, the value and importance of recognition of their own suffering and emotional state, and at least some acknowledgement that the very suffering experienced was a result of valuable relationships (for them, and for patients/families). As suggested earlier, one interesting outcome of the battle these doctors had with their own emotions was the tendency to hand over 'sentimental work' to nurses, a (still) largely female workforce (Kirby et al., 2014).

Nursing, dying and (gendered) emotions at work

It is impossible to consider inter-professional relations between medicine and nursing without also considering the (evolving) gendered division of labour within hospital settings. Whilst the nursing profession has shifted dramatically over the past few decades in terms of its profile and practice, there are distinctly gendered dimensions to the emotional work of healthcare professions (Gray, 2010; Henderson, 2001). It is still relatively easy to see the links between ideas about 'women's work' and nursing work, and the emotional components of care within clinical settings (Bolton, 2001; McQueen, 2004; Mok & Chiu, 2004; Skilbeck & Payne, 2003). Contribution to, experience of, and engagement in, forms of suffering should thus in turn be viewed as embedded in such historical and culturally-located gender dynamics (Broom et al., 2015) and contemporary logics of professional roles (e.g. nurses as involved in 'care', doctors as involved in 'treatment', women as more 'caring', men as more 'cognitive/rational') (Hochschild, 1983, 1979; Ungerson, 2006). While such logics are often strongly contested, and are erroneous in practice, they are nevertheless important for understanding the historical, political and cultural context of these professions. Indeed, some of the nurses interviewed were men, and many of the doctors interviewed were women. However, there remains a gendered context to the role, regardless of the gendered 'make up' of the professionals. Nursing work was (and for some, and in some cultural contexts still is) synonymous with 'women's work' (Bolton, 2001; Broom et al., 2016). Any reading of affective dimensions of labour and experiencing suffering therein must thus acknowledge this cultural history and the relegation of feelings to women in fields that have traditionally been female-dominated (for example, nursing, social work, childcare). The following data is situated within this historical and professional context, and thus should be concurrently read as shaped by both gendered and nurse-medical relations. Within the interviews, the nurses were much clearer on the emotional impact of their role in contexts of futility, transition to palliative care, and the dying process. These nurses reflected on their own (often acute) suffering, that of the patient and family, and their crucial role therein:

Tracey: There's every emotion you could think of, you know sometimes it's just business as usual because we do a lot of palliation here . . . we see a lot of death on this ward, so that's not too terrifying for the nurses usually . . . like it's never, it's never easy, but you get, you learn, develop coping mechanisms, I guess, as you get older, or as you've worked longer in nursing to deal with the things that happen every day. . . . It's not the patients that is the saddest, hardest thing, it's the relatives grieving that is the hardest thing to cope with . . . I think the nurses focus in a way on the tasks that we need to do. It doesn't mean they don't see the person that's going through it, but it just does allow you to cope if you know that you're giving as much as you can by making it as easy as you can for that patient, if that makes sense. [Nurse, Female]

Interviewer: How do you feel about telling people 'you're going to die?' And having that discussion, how do you personally feel about that?

Kat: Sometimes, yeah, sometimes I do take it home. Sometimes I do . . . We've had a young lady just recently, a 50-year-old, who has breast cancer, who now has brain [metastases]. She's been very difficult on the ward, and we had a family meeting last week. And I swear, there was 20 members of the family and probably six staff, and we were all in tears when we came out, every one of us . . . In the middle of the meeting she kept going 'why me? why me?' and screaming . . . It's very difficult, you're telling these people she's got weeks to live. [Nurse, Female]

Audrey: Look, the end-of-life stuff I think is not great . . . I mean we often try and get people [to have] debriefings and stuff like that. But they normally turn out to be fizzers, [nurses] don't want to talk in front of people . . . some of the younger girls seem to be better at that. They like to cry then and there, and I think that's probably a good thing . . . then other people just want to dash to their car and just go, and I think the moment's lost then. [Nurse, Female]

The nurses' accounts provide a nuanced, but still often problematic, view of the place of feelings within their everyday work, involving, just as the doctors', a tussle around what is acceptable to express, to feel, to engage with in their professional lives (Froggatt, 1998). It was clear in the interviews that the nurses experienced considerable suffering – within the nursing–patient–family relation – and that to some extent this was considered an expected and normal aspect of nursing work. Yet, there was also a strong desire to 'run away' and 'deal with it' (or suffer) in private. The nurses felt that they were expected to take on the sentimental aspects of care within this context, and it is revealing that the nurses continue to refer to colleagues as 'girls', despite some nurses (albeit a minority) being men. While on one level reflective of the gendered nature of the cohort, it is also revealing that 'young girls' were considered best at expressiveness, and the senior nurses considered themselves less able to express emotions in the workplace. This is likely to reflect the gendered character of seniority and the required performances within professional hierarchies (and the emphasis on normative masculine characteristics of control/repression) (Bell et al., 2014; Gray, 2010; McQueen, 2004).

Moreover, the above accounts demonstrate the need felt by nurses to bracket emotions and reduce experiences of, or indeed repress, suffering over time, in order to prevent professional burnout (however contradictory this may read from a psychoanalytic perspective). The nurses valued 'sitting in the moment' with emotions, processing their own personal grief and sense of loss as patients died or were referred to end-of-life care. The nurses accepted that while dying was 'business as usual', it took a significant emotional toll, and they recognised that they were suffering alongside patients. This was vastly different to how the doctors articulated and made sense of their therapeutic encounters and the affective dimensions of treatment and care. Still, the nurses in turn articulated the importance of emotion management, and the precariousness of emotions as professional competence vis-à-vis 'letting them too close'. A common reflection was that the (also gendered) dynamic of being involved in 'rescuing' was difficult to avoid, but that it nevertheless needed to be 'reined in':

Eileen: . . . the partners, the wives, the husbands . . . quite often they'll come in and sit in the seat and cry their eyes out. 'How am I going to tell our children? What's the best way of telling our children? How am I going to tell his mother?' They're at a total loss . . . I'm thinking 'oh god, I've got ten minutes' . . . But you don't want that person to think they're not getting 100 per cent from you. [But] . . . I can't go around rescuing people. I don't want come off as a rescuer . . . [Nurse, Female]

Jody: . . . nursing's a hard balance . . . There's always something in every person's life there is always something horrible or something difficult that we've had to deal with, whether it's in healthcare that often our patients will bring back to us. It's just, I guess, a skill that you learn as you go along as to how to deal with it. [Nurse]

Kate: It's hard not to be involved. But to the same extent, I don't think I can do my best if I'm overly involved with them, with my emotions. [Nurse, Female]

Normalising sentimentality: 'close enough, but not too close'

There is a rich body of work within the social sciences on intimacy, sentimentality and emotion in nursing work (Bolton, 2001; Henderson, 2001; Hochschild, 1979; Phillips, 1996; Theodosius, 2006); indeed, the nurse–patient relationship is one that is recognised as involving intimacy, touch and emotional engagement; nurses *access* suffering, grief and trauma more acutely than many medical staff (Ablett & Jones, 2007; Field, 1989; Fillion et al., 2007; Sandgren et al., 2006). Being present at the bedside, for example, places nurses in a context whereby the hour-by-hour, day-by-day undulations of disease progression and human suffering are dominant within their professional milieu (Morris & Thomas, 2007; Morita et al., 2004; Skilbeck & Payne, 2003). They are subsumed within the collective atmosphere of grief, hope, loss, anger, rage and melancholia.

Moreover, as opposed to the context of doctors, managing and displaying feelings is a core (recognised) skill in the work of nurses. A lack of (albeit restrained) emotions is perceived as poor professional competence. The sense of 'balance' of professionalism versus sentimentality is thus different than for medicine, as is the *expression of*, and willingness to *sit with*, suffering. The nurses interviewed felt able to acknowledge emotions, the blurring of the personal and professional ('they remind me of dad'), and the importance of such dynamics for relationships and their everyday work:

Interviewer: And what happens [when people get to you]?
Trish: Then you go home and cry and move on for another day . . . it's not a mistake [to feel], it's something that you do. You'll always have someone that'll jump in under that [emotional] barrier sort of thing. . . . you might say 'oh, they remind me of my sister', or 'they remind me of dad', or whatever sort of thing. We've all done it, but it's being able to cut yourself back off from, and not getting, getting close enough but not too close. [Nurse, Female]

Rebecca:	I think you can't treat every patient as your best friend. At the end of the day, it's our job. But there are some that sneak through the cracks who sort of get to you. [Nurse, Female]
Angela:	But it's got to be this balance between being resilient and still caring deeply about things. [Nurse, Female]
Alexandra:	. . . you've known these people and their family for years usually, and it's really hard. And you go home feeling you know, you do, you go off and have a little sook [cry]. And the way I cope is, I do a lot of exercise and it just works, you clear your head, you go for a run. And then you come home and you just say 'hello everyone'. 'How was your day?' 'It was tough, it was really tough. Today I lost someone who was really important to me.' . . . it would be unrealistic to expect that it's not going to be tough, you know what I mean? You know what's going to happen in this job. And it doesn't make you tougher or get this thick skin, because we're generally, I think, as a group of people [nurses are] probably more sensitive than most because you know, [nurses] we're sookies [sic]. But a good cry doesn't hurt . . . [Nurse, Female]

The nurses recognised that managing emotions within the hospital was delegated to them (often as women, although not always, but certainly as *nurses* vis-à-vis doctors) and that this was both a professional skill as well as a personal challenge (see also Li, 2004; Li & Arber, 2006). Thus, they aimed to create a careful balance between relations of care, and not inducing too much suffering on their part as nurses. They recognised and reflected on their interpersonal boundary work, and forms of self-protection. They also reflected on their role in accommodating doctors' desires to avoid their own emotions and forms of suffering therein, and the implications for all stakeholders:

Talia:	So the way it tends to happen around here is the oncologist or the haematologist comes in with very little tact often, delivers bad news, paints a very grim picture of things and then says palliative care will come and see you. So, often the first consultation you have with the patient they're like deer in the headlights, 'oh my god palliative care are here, I've been told it's all bad news you know, what's the next step?' And you're sort of backpedalling . . . it's presented [by the doctor] as a choice to the patient, as if 'you've failed' you know? [Nurse, Female]
Lynda:	I think partly because some [doctors] don't like talking about death, like it's not part of a conversation that they probably have the comfort to have or the skills to have . . . That's a much easier conversation. I think sometimes it just comes down to the [specialist] just doesn't know how to do it. [Nurse, Female]
Anna:	. . . it all swings on the physician conversations. And how the physicians have communicated with the patients . . . it can be a whole lot better if the physician is just really honest and upfront with the patient. You

know, some of them do it beautifully, but some of them don't do it at all because it's a hard conversation to have, and that makes it really hard for the nurses. You know, sometimes we've got patients who you know have metastatic disease, absolutely zero chance of survival, and yet we are still doing active treatments. And that just sends a very conflicted message to the patient. [Nurse, Female]

Above, we can see that emotions matter within the therapeutic encounter, and are complicit in the trajectories of patients (toward palliative or end-of-life care), but also in the work of other professionals. Moreover, the avoidance of grief, sadness, suffering and so forth – or complex affective dimensions of illness and care – on the part of some professionals (mostly doctors) meant that patients themselves stayed on what the nurses often regarded as futile treatment. That is, the relational desire for optimism (Li, 2004) and the desire to avoid collective suffering, functions to prevent transparency within the therapeutic encounter. Affective denialism is thus enmeshed in collective suffering. This points to the need to explore how the practices of medicine and nursing are embedded in the acceptance (or lack thereof) of human suffering, and that a patient's supposed suffering (from cancer or another condition) is in turn shaped by the inter-subjective, and cultural taboos around death, dying and bereavement (McNamara et al., 1995; Meyer, 1995; Willmott, 2000). Moreover, these dynamics are embedded in various professional projects, jurisdictions (medicine as 'disease beaters', nurses as 'sentimental workers') and moral structures that purport the value of illness and wellness as tied to will.

Therapeutic encounters and treatment trajectories as collective suffering

We are not the first researchers to consider the role and impact of emotions within medicine and nursing. In fact, there has been considerable attention paid to this issue, although largely from a descriptive/empirical position (Abendroth & Flannery, 2006; Potter et al., 2010; Sprang et al., 2007). Yet, hitherto research in this area has treated emotions-at-work in a simplistic fashion – to be managed, limited, controlled or side-lined – or to be considered as a site for training and professional education. Rather, we understand these moments as affective assemblages, produced through such things as professional projects, cultural taboos, therapeutic alliances, resistance to mortality and the repression of feelings. As outlined in the Introduction, while a reductive analysis outlines a discrete sufferer and carer subject position, a more nuanced analysis reveals how lines become blurred, with a relational ontology necessary to explore how affective relations are co-produced, move across bodies and persons, and create (and are created by) atmospheres of pain, hope, guilt, resilience, recovery and persistence. We also view these narratives as providing important insights into how suffering is 'treated' in caring relations. Where is it perceived as being located and for what reasons? We would argue that hitherto a one-directional model has dominated (cared for/caring; caring/suffering), concealing the true experience of professional practice and collective suffering.

This concealment of the collective experience of (professional/collective) suffering has pernicious effects. It conceals the very ambitions, desires and contributions clinicians make to a patient and their suffering. It conceals clinicians *wanting* things to be, *willing* things to happen, and *desiring* particular outcomes. Finally, the concrete actions that clinicians may take to achieve a desirable outcome (to just 'press on' regardless, to 'try something' else, to not 'give up') are also concealed. None of this has made it into the current scholarly understandings of the dynamics of suffering at the end of life. Yet we know that optimism (as affect) is enmeshed with (denial of) futility, and that 'holding onto hope' can be both productive and detrimental (see also Ahmed, 2004). We seek not to assess what it is, but rather, to emphasise that such things are part of the affective relations and can contribute to suffering therein. Further, we seek to demonstrate that suffering is not merely emotional, but bio-physical, embodied, spiritual, cultural and so forth (if one can meaningfully separate out facets of suffering). We seek to demonstrate that 'non-patient' subjects can feel suffering *in their bodies.*

We also posit that suffering as currently conceived – *as emergent specifically and exclusively from the (dying) person* – evades the everyday practice of professionals offering a gift of care, but also, practising its removal (see also Back et al., 2009). As evident in some of the doctors' accounts, they simply 'don't care' in order to avoid affective complexities. There is, of course, a certain grief embedded within this withdrawal – sometimes from clinician and patient, and sometimes only from clinician. Forms of emotion management that were talked about in the interviews included dissociation and detachment may also be an articulation (or indeed outcome) of suffering. Suffering and subsequent relations of care thus operate as a collective atmosphere with actions and reactions emergent from them. Clinicians, whatever their position on emotional engagement, offer their own loss, grief and disappointment to the therapeutic dynamic, and this in turn shapes the overall trajectory of care. The critical nature of awareness of this dynamic is that such emotions may dictate when active treatment will stop and when patients are 'allowed' to let go. Placing this in the context of an existing scholarly literature which thoroughly (over) emphasises the dying person's suffering (i.e. 'total pain', 'denial'), there is a need to explore the emotional world of clinicians, and its intersections with other life worlds, emotions and affective practices. One could imagine how patient complicity in the avoiding of grief on the part of the doctor, for instance, would feed into existing normative constructs surrounding cancer patients, in particular. As Steinberg notes:

> The assertion of this subject doubly crowds out her obverse – the bad patient, she who might not be interested in marching forward (or be able to do so), who might not be invested in life at any cost, or perhaps even at all, she who is 'not brave' – and indeed, what does a 'not brave' cancer patient look like?
>
> (2015, p. 35)

A lack of acknowledgment of dying, the pursuit of optimism, hope and 'marching forward' (see Chapter 6 for an exploration of patient perspectives on this dynamic), may be intimately enmeshed in the professionals' underlying grief and resistance to failure (and in turn, the patients' willingness to submit to such normative notions) (Zimmermann, 2007).

Thus, we argue for two shifts in thinking around this area of care. The first involves acknowledging the affective dimensions that professionals contribute to (and that people are drawn to). The second shift involves understanding the notion of suffering at the end of life as an affective assemblage, inter-subjectively constructed, technologically mediated, and reflecting tussles between professional projects, individual ambitions, cultural taboos and embodied experiences. Suffering, we posit, lies across these spheres and actors. The dynamic of 'holding on' to cancer patients, for example by many doctors, or by the dogged pursuit of so-called 'active treatment' (rather than the timely shift to life enhancing treatment) may be a manifestation of such emotional moments and intersections. That is, care is shaped by the desires and needs of the clinician, many of which emerge from sites of suffering which often go unacknowledged (or are delegated to other actors such as nurses). Further work is needed to explore health professionals' attempts to balance their own emotions and sentimentality versus their performance of expertise and professionalism. This assemblage emerges from desire: desire on the part of the doctor to fix; desire of the nurse to care; desire from the patient's carer for longevity or for the fight to end; desire from the patient for many things, including comfort, quality, relief, hope, longevity or brevity. Patient desire has been examined to the point where it is almost exclusively their emotions which are used to make sense of what occurs. Yet, it is often the *desires* of other stakeholders, including doctors and nurses (in conjunction with those of patients and families) that shape the trajectory of engagement with technologies, and the perpetuation of or amelioration of suffering. In effect, we are suggesting that emotions are not (and should not be) relegated to a suffering patient; everyone is part of the assemblage, and although not equal contributors, they are contributors nonetheless. One does not need to be ill or dying to be part of, or even crucial to, suffering. In fact, seemingly peripheral actors may be merely concealed from their role in the affective atmospheres which fundamentally *make up* experiences of hope, loss, grief, acceptance, and hopelessness (among many others).

Finally, it is worth emphasising the gendered problematic of sentimental work being allocated to nurses, and largely (although not exclusively) to women within the professional sphere. Whilst it may indeed be the case – as the accounts presented indicate – that nurses both facilitate and manage emotional expression in the wards, acting as *intimate* mediators, such dynamics are problematic on numerous levels. The first problematic dynamic is the concealment of the emotional drivers of the doctor–patient dynamic. This concealment is built on the assumption that emotions are compartmentalised and that the medical encounter (or, perhaps more accurately, the doctor) is objective and rational, rather than emotive and driven by feelings. This is clearly not the case as doctors (varyingly) report being highly influenced by their emotions.

The second problematic dynamic involves how sentimental work has been complicit in the perpetuation of medical dominance. As Strauss (1978) points out in his classic analysis of nurse–medical relations, maintaining the sentimental order of the hospital is reflective of the protection of a historical gendered division of labour between nursing (care) and medicine (science). The denial of *the relation* of suffering with therapeutic relationships – and its gendered mediations – creates an erroneous picture of affective assemblages within the hospital. Unpacking affective entanglements (both acknowledged and denied) is an important aspect of understanding (and even reducing) the multifaceted experience of suffering within this and other clinical contexts.

Note

1 For an analysis of what counts as a 'good' or 'liveable' life, see Butler (2000).

References

Abendroth, M. & Flannery, J. (2006). Predicting the risk of compassion fatigue: A study of hospice nurses. *Journal of Hospice & Palliative Nursing*, 8(6), pp. 346–356.

Ablett, J. R. & Jones, R. (2007). Resilience and well-being in palliative care staff. *Psycho-Oncology*, 16(8), pp. 733–40.

Adamle, K. & Ludwick, R. (2005). Humor in hospice care: Who, where, and how much? *American Journal of Hospice & Palliative Care*, 22(4), pp. 287–290.

Ahmed, S. (2004). Collective feelings or, the impressions left by others. *Theory, Culture & Society*, 21(2), pp. 25–42.

Ahmed, S. (2010). *The Promise of Happiness.* Durham, NC: Duke University Press.

Back, A. L., Young, J. P., McCown, E., Engelberg, R. A., Vig, E. K., Reinke, L. F. & Curtis, J. R. (2009) Abandonment at the end of life from patient, caregiver, nurse, and physician perspectives. *Archives of Internal Medicine*, 169(5), pp. 474–479.

Bailey, C., Murphy, R. & Porock, D. (2011). Professional tears: Developing emotional intelligence around death and dying in emergency work. *Journal of Clinical Nursing*, 20(23–24), pp. 3364–3372.

Bell, A. V., Michalec, B. & Arenson, C. (2014). The (stalled) progress of interprofessional collaboration: the role of gender. *Journal of Interprofessional Care*, 28(2), pp. 98–102.

Bendelow, G. & Williams, S. J., eds. (1998). *Emotions in Social Life: Critical Themes and Contemporary Issues.* London: Routledge

Bolton, S. (2001). Changing faces: Nurses as emotional jugglers. *Sociology of Health & Illness*, 23(1), pp. 85–100.

Boston, P., Bruce, A. & Schreiber, R. (2011). Existential suffering in the palliative care setting: An integrated literature review. *Journal of Pain and Symptom Management*, 41(3), pp. 604–618.

Broom, A. (2015). *Dying: A Social Perspective on the End of Life.* Ashgate: Farnham.

Broom, A. & Kirby, E. (2013). The end of life and the family: Hospice patients' views on dying as relational. *Sociology of Health and Illness*, 35(4), pp. 499–513.

Broom, A., Kirby, E., Adams, J. & Refshauge, K. (2015). On illegitimacy, suffering and recognition: A diary study of women living with chronic pain. *Sociology*, 49(4), pp. 712–773.

Broom, A., Kirby, E., Good, P. & Lwin, Z. (2016). Nursing futility, managing medicine: Nurses' perspectives on the transition from life-prolonging to palliative care. *Health*, 20(6), 653–670.

Broom, A., Kirby, E., Good, P., Wootton, J. & Adams, J. (2014). The troubles of telling: Managing communication about the end of life. *Qualitative Health Research*, 24(2), pp. 151–162.

Broom, A., Kirby, E., Good, P., Wootton, J. & Adams, J. (2013). The art of letting go: Referral to palliative care and its discontents. *Social Science and Medicine*, 78, pp. 9–16.

Broom, A., Kirby, E., Good, P., Wootton, J., Hardy, J. & Yates, P. (2014). Negotiating futility, managing emotions: Nursing the transition to palliative care. *Qualitative Health Research*, 25(3), pp. 299–309.

Broom, A., Wong, T., Kirby, E., Harrup, Karikios, R. & Lwin, Z. (2016). A qualitative study of medical oncologists' experiences of their profession and workforce sustainability. *PLOS ONE*, 11(11), e0166302.

Brown, R., Dunn, S., Byrnes, K., Morris, R., Heinrich, P. & Shaw, J. (2009). Doctors' stress responses and poor communication performance in simulated bad-news consultations. *Academic Medicine*, 84(11), pp. 1595–1602.

Butler, J. (2000). *Frames of War: When is Life Grievable?* London, New York: Verso.

Chattoo, S. & Ahmad, W. I. (2008). The moral economy of selfhood and caring. *Sociology of Health & Illness*, 30(4), pp. 550–564.

Cheng, J., Lo, R. & Woo, J. (2013) Anticipatory grief therapy for older persons nearing the end of life. *Aging Health*, 9(1), pp. 103–114.

Denier, Y., Dierckx de Casterlé, B., De Bal, N. & Gastmans, C. (2010). 'It's intense, you know': Nurses' experiences in caring for patients requesting euthanasia. *Medicine, Health Care & Philosophy*, 13(1), pp. 41–48.

Dragojlovic, A. (2015). Affective geographies: Intergenerational hauntings, bodily affectivity and multiracial subjectivities. *Subjectivity*, 8(4), pp. 315–334.

Field, D. (1989). *Nursing the Dying*. London: Tavistock/Routledge.

Fillion, L., Tremblay, I., Truchon, M., Côté, D., Struthers, C. W. & Dupuis, R. (2007). Job satisfaction and emotional distress among nurses providing palliative care. *International Journal of Stress Management*, 14(1), pp. 1–25.

Fox, J. (2006). 'Notice how you feel': An alternative to detached concern among hospice volunteers. *Qualitative Health Research*, 16(7), pp. 944–961.

Fox, R. C. & Lief, H. (1963). Training for 'detached concern'. In H. Lief, ed., *The Psychological Basis of Medical Practice*. New York, NY: Harper & Row, pp. 12–35.

Friedrichsen, M. & Strang, P. (2003). Doctors' strategies when breaking bad news to terminally ill patients. *Journal of Palliative Medicine*, 6(4), pp. 565–574.

Froggatt, K. (1998). The place of metaphor and language in exploring nurses' emotional work. *Journal of Advanced Nursing*, 28(2), pp. 332–338.

Graham, R. (2006). Lacking compassion: Sociological analyses of the medical profession. *Social Theory & Health*, 4(1), pp. 43–63.

Gray, B. (2010). Emotional labour, gender and professional stereotypes of emotional and physical contact, and personal perspectives on the emotional labour of nursing. *Journal of Gender Studies*, 19(4), pp. 349–360.

Henderson, A. (2001). Emotional labor and nursing: An under-appreciated aspect of caring work. *Nursing Inquiry*, 8(2), pp. 130–138.

Hochschild, A. (1979). Emotion work, feeling rules, and social structure. *American Journal of Sociology*, 85(3), pp. 551–575.

Hochschild, A. (1983). *The Managed Heart*. Berkeley, CA: University of California Press.

Kellehear, A. (1984). Are we a death denying society? A sociological review. *Social Science and Medicine*, 18(9), pp. 713–723.

Kirby, E., Broom, A. & Good, P. (2014) The role and significance of nurses in managing transitions to palliative care: A qualitative study. *BMJ Open*, 4, DOI: 10.1136/bmjopen-2014–006026

Li, S. (2004) 'Symbiotic niceness': Constructing a therapeutic relationship in psychosocial palliative care. *Social Science & Medicine*, 58(12), pp. 2571–2583.

Li, S. & Arber, A. (2006) The construction of troubled and credible patients: A study of emotion talk in palliative care settings. *Qualitative Health Research*, 16, pp. 27–46.

MacArtney, J., Broom, A., Kirby, E., Good, P. & Wootton, J. (2017). The liminal and the parallax: Living and dying at the end of life. *Qualitative Health Research*, 27(5), pp. 623–633, DOI: 10.1177/1049732315618938.

MacArtney, J., Broom, A., Kirby, E., Good, P., Wootton, J. & Adams, J. (2015). On resilience and acceptance in the transition to palliative care at the end of life. *Health*, 19(3), pp. 263–279.

MacArtney, J., Broom, A., Kirby, E., Good, P., Wootton, J. & Adams, J. (2016). Locating care at the end of life: Burden, vulnerability, and the practical accomplishment of dying. *Sociology of Health and Illness*, 38(3), pp. 479–492.

McNamara, B., Waddell, C. & Colvin, M. (1995). Threats to the good death: The cultural context of stress and coping among hospice nurses. *Sociology of Health & Illness*, 17(2), pp. 222–241.

McQueen, A. C. (2004). Emotional intelligence in nursing work. *Journal of Advanced Nursing*, 47(1), pp. 101–108.

McSteen, K. & Peden-McAlpine, C. (2006). The role of the nurse as advocate in ethically difficult care situations with dying patients. *Journal of Hospice & Palliative Nursing*, 8(5), pp. 259–269.

Melvin, S. & Oldham, L. (2009). When to refer patients to palliative care: Triggers, traps and timely referrals. *Journal of Hospice & Palliative Nursing*, 11(5), pp. 291–301.

Meyer, M. (1995) Dignity, death and modern virtue. *American Philosophical Quarterly*, 32(1), pp. 45–56.

Miller, K. L., Reeves, S., Zwarenstein, M., Beales, J. D., Kenaszchuk, C. & Conn, L. G. (2008). Nursing emotion work and inter-professional collaboration in general internal medicine wards: A qualitative study. *Journal of Advanced Nursing*, 64(4): 332–343.

Mok, E. & Chiu, P. C. (2004). Nurse–patient relationships in palliative care. *Journal of Advanced Nursing*, 48(5), pp. 475–483.

Mol, A. (2008). *The Logic of Care*. Abingdon, Oxon: Routledge.

Morita, T., Miyashita, M., Kimura, R., Adachi, I. & Shima, Y. (2004). Emotional burden of nurses in palliative sedation therapy. *Palliative Medicine*, 18(6): 550–557.

Morris, S. M. & Thomas, C. (2007). Placing the dying body: Emotional, situational and embodied factors in preferences for place of final care and death in cancer. In Davidson, J., Bondi, L. & Smith, M., eds, *Emotional Geographies*. Aldershot, England: Taylor & Francis, pp. 19–31.

Nettleton, S., Burrows, R. & Watt, I. (2008). How do you feel Doctor? An analysis of emotional aspects of routine professional medical work. *Social Theory & Health*, 6(1), pp. 18–36.

Nielsen, M. K., Neergaard, M. A., Jensen, A. B., Bro, F. & Guldin, M. B. (2016). Do we need to change our understanding of anticipatory grief in caregivers? A systematic review of caregiver studies during end-of-life caregiving and bereavement. *Clinical Psychology Review*, 44, pp. 75–93.

Phillips, S. (1996) Labouring the emotions: Expanding the remit of nursing work? *Journal of Advanced Nursing*, 24(1), pp. 139–143.

Potter, P., Deshields, T., Divanbeigi, J., Berger, J. & Cipriano, D. (2010) Compassion fatigue and burnout: Prevalence among oncology nurses. *Clinical Journal of Oncology Nursing*, 14(5), pp. E56–62.

Sandgren, A., Thulesius, H., Fridlund, B. & Petersson, K. (2006). Striving for emotional survival in palliative cancer nursing. *Qualitative Health Research*, 16(1), pp. 79–96.

Skilbeck, J. & Payne, S. (2003) Emotional support and the role of clinical nurse specialists in palliative care. *Journal of Advanced Nursing*, 43(5), pp. 521–530.

Slocum-Gori, S., Hemsworth, D., Chan, W. W., Carson, A. & Kazanjian, A. (2013). Understanding compassion satisfaction, compassion fatigue and burnout: A survey of the hospice palliative care workforce. *Palliative Medicine*, 27(2), pp. 172–178.

Smith, C., Nelson, J., Berman, A., Powell, C., Fleischman, J., Salazar-Schicchi, J. & Wisnivesky, J. (2012). Lung cancer physicians' referral practices for palliative care consultation. *Annals of Oncology*, 23(2), pp. 382–387.

Sprang, G., Clark, J. J. & Whitt-Woosley, A. (2007). Compassion fatigue, compassion satisfaction, and burnout: Factors impacting a professional's quality of life. *Journal of Loss and Trauma*, 12(3), pp. 259–280.

Steinberg, D. (2015) The bad patient: Estranged subjects of the cancer culture. *Body & Society*, 2(3), pp. 115–143.

Strauss, A. L. (1978). *Negotiations: Varieties, Contexts, Processes and Social Order*. London: Jossey-Bass.

Sweeting, H. N. & Gilhooly, M. L. M. (1990). Anticipatory grief: A review. *Social Science and Medicine*, 30(10), pp. 1073–1080.

Temel, J., Greer, J., Muzikansky, A., Gallagher, E., Admane, S., Jackson, V. et al. (2010). Early palliative care for patients with metastatic non-small-cell lung cancer. *The New England Journal of Medicine*, 363(8), pp. 733–742.

The, A., Hak, T., Koeter, G. & van Der Wal, G. (2000). Collusion in doctor–patient communication about imminent death: An ethnographic study. *British Medical Journal*, 321, pp. 1376–1381.

Theodosius, C. (2006). Recovering emotion from emotion management. *Sociology*, 40(5), pp. 893–910.

Ungerson C. (2006) Care, work and feeling. *The Sociological Review*, 54, pp. 188–203.

Willmott, H. (2000). Death. So what? Sociology, sequestration and emancipation. *The Sociological Review*, 48(4), pp. 649–665.

Zimmermann, C. (2007) Death denial: Obstacle or instrument for palliative care? An analysis of clinical literature. *Sociology of Health & Illness*, 29(2), pp. 297–314.

Zimmermann, C. (2012). Acceptance of dying: A discourse analysis of palliative care literature. *Social Science & Medicine*, 75(1), pp. 217–224.

2 A labour of love?

Suffering in relation in informal care for the dying

Introduction

> [Palliative care] should be care of the person . . . that is dying but also care of their immediate family. That is what a lot of people forget. Because [people] are so caught up in the person that is actually dying . . .
>
> [Carer]

Confronting our own death, or the death of people we are close to, is one of the most challenging personal and interpersonal moments we will face across the life course (Broom, 2015). While death may not always be physically painful, untimely or even sad, the dying process is usually emotionally and interpersonally intense and often challenging for the many participants in the dying process. Actor and director Orson Welles famously stated that 'we're born alone, we live alone, we die alone; only through our love and friendship can we create the illusion for the moment that we're not alone.' This neatly captures the broader cultural tendency to construe dying in highly individualised terms. Suffering therein – whether emotional, spiritual or physical – becomes necessarily located within the individual who is dying (Beck & Beck-Gernsheim, 1996; West, 2002). Carer suffering is, in turn, often bracketed off – the *bereavement period* being a good example – offering time-limited stage for carers' and families' suffering post-death (Doka, 2002).

While dying certainly has individualised facets – and there is often an ensuing existential, individualised crisis in the dying process – sentiments such as those described above lack an understanding of how dying and suffering is highly relational (Broom & Kirby, 2013); and how the dying person is entwined with, and connected to, other persons, bodies, techniques and practices. Whether in relation to formalised care (see Chapter 1) or informal care, dying is necessarily about interpersonal entanglement, affective tussles, and suffering *within* and often *because of* forms of relationality. The individualisation of suffering, for those who are dying and for those who are caring for the dying, has created a problematic series of logics around who is 'facing death', 'feeling pain', 'suffering loss' and 'experiencing grief'. Such logics have evaded the reality that suffering during the dying process necessarily moves across people, families and carers (both informal and formal as shown in Chapters 1 and 6) (Broom & Kirby, 2013); it is circulating, difficult to pin down and settles on (and is bolstered by) people.

In this chapter, we seek to articulate how *dying and suffering are shared* between the person at the end of their life, people, children, partners and friends. We also seek to raise questions about the affective dimensions of caring, challenge simplistic assumptions about who is suffering and the purpose of care, and how 'caring relations' can be experienced as suffering in and of themselves. The tendency to conceive of suffering in the dying process in individualised terms suggests the need to consider how the lived experience of caring for the dying may illustrate a different *ontology of suffering* (cf. Chattoo and Ahmad, 2008). The importance of such an understanding is heightened by the fact that individualised models are imbued in and by medical interventions; the concepts of individualised pain and symptom management (Broom & Kirby, 2013) and or 'carer supportive care needs' (Arksey and Glendinning, 2007; Harding & Higginson, 2001). While important for dealing with the physical specificities of dying, such categorisations evade the dyadic character of suffering within the dying process, and likely reduce capacity to address complex relational sufferings within the dying process (Burns et al., 2015; Chattoo and Ahmad, 2008; MacArtney et al., 2017).

In returning to the overarching theme of this book, this chapter explores caring for the dying as a critical example of *suffering in/as relation*. The focus here then is on the key aspects of (relational) suffering that carers perceive, experience and are part of the *production of*. While Chapter 1 explored the complicity, investment and experience of doctors and nurses of suffering in the context of futility and the end of life in relation, this chapter reveals a range of relational, inter-subjective experiences also often concealed within healthcare settings and indeed the dying process. These include what carers experience in terms of emotions and suffering therein during the end of life. One important reason that the experiences and suffering of informal carers (family, partners, friends and 'significant others') has been largely overlooked is the cultural reification of the moral and ethical value of informal care (Fisher & Tronto, 1990; Held, 2006; Tronto, 1993, 1998). In talking about an ethic of care, we tend to conceive care as an offering from one person to another, in turn (potentially) reinforcing the notion of individualised suffering.

In this chapter, we seek a reorientation of suffering across actors. Just as the professional values of objectivity, mastery and benevolence conceal professional suffering in Chapter 1, the normativities of informing caring relations (including the cultural value of care as gift and sacrifice) push suffering into problematic territory. For example, the 'labour' of caring, in colloquial terms, is often viewed as a *'labour of love'*, yet the affective dimensions of caring relations (in this context, at the end of life) are much more untidy and relational than this. As we shall show, positive affective dimensions can be completely absent; yet this is rarely discussed in relation to care for the dying. Caring for the dying, whether as a partner, child, parent, family member or friend, is a challenging and often conflicted series of progressively difficult moments, conjuring up many competing affective relations, including moralities of gift and sacrifice, and relational demands including hope, stoicism, optimism, dependency and so on (Twigg & Atkin, 1994; West, 2002). Yet rarely in the academic literature have the relations of suffering for the carer (in relation) been explored, particularly in end-of-life contexts. We posit here that informal care for the dying brings with it considerable relational suffering across family units and social relations, and this interpersonal affective dimension is often side-lined due to the perception of the experience of the 'dying person' and (soon-to-be) 'bereaved carer'. Waiting until the point of bereavement to acknowledge suffering (and allowing affective negativity), and the complexity of caring relations, is an inadequate and potentially harmful approach.

Care as connected bodies, techniques and practices

The sensibility of dying as the ultimate individualised act is a common misunderstanding of the (relational) experience, meaning and acts of dying. This relates to the understanding of what care (and thus a 'carer' role) is in this and in other healthcare contexts (Held, 2006; Kittay, 1999; Thomas et al., 2002; Tronto, 1993; 1998; Twigg & Atkin, 1994; West, 2002). The sensibility of dying raises once again the questions (posed in our Introduction and elsewhere in this book) as what constitutes a relation of care, whether this relation of care moves in particular directions (cared for, carer), and what it achieves and means for different people located (and its relation to suffering). Moreover, a key dynamic in the broader scholarly work on care has been to examine how informal care as a cultural and social *practice* functions for individuals, families, communities and nations (Chattoo & Ahmad, 2008). This has involved critical analysis of 'informal care' as an action, something delivered, received or provided, but more helpfully, 'care' as reflective of various connectivities between people, bodies and practices (Held, 2005; Tronto, 1993; 1998; Twigg & Atkin, 1994).

Furthermore, care can be seen as the articulation of (culturally located) moral and ethical agreements between people, families and citizens. This includes an understanding that we 'care' as *affective entanglement* (i.e. because of such things as intimacy, love, affection) but also out of *structural necessity* (i.e. collective 'insurance' for survival or as part of the social contract around rights and responsibilities for mutual benefit). This involves the (temporal) allocation of roles that *produce* distinct carer and caring identities and categories, despite being in fact diffuse, co-located and blurred in practice. Relations of care are thus political, historical and economic entities, produced by evolving and culturally-located social norms, concurrently articulating the (often gendered) politics of gift/sacrifice, duty/obligation, citizenship/rights, survival/resilience (Bailey & Robertson, 2015; Bauman 1991; Berecki-Gisolf et al., 2008; Bubeck 1995).

Caring relations are also boundary-crossing, with the dynamics of pain and suffering (more on this below) moving across, being shared by, and co-produced by the range of actors involved in dying, including carers and health professionals (MacArtney et al., 2017; Thomas et al., 2002). Pain is shared – it is not located within a person or persons; rather the act of care and suffering therein is a relational practice. Whilst in this chapter we focus on carers' perspectives, their accounts also reveal that many of the assumed logics of caring/being cared for/ being a carer are unsettled. Moreover, carers' own experiences of suffering (in relation) shows the ways in which dying is in fact shared as a moment across people. This has implications for our understanding of the dynamics of suffering at the end of life and more broadly. First, a 'hangover' from previous misunderstandings of care – as gift, giving, offering, directional – rather than co-located across people – means that the experiences of carer suffering (in relation) have been sidelined. The prioritisation of suffering as individualised has also meant that institutional practices (i.e. in hospitals and hospice), the dynamics of place (i.e. dying at home versus hospice), the limits of biomedical intervention (i.e. what can, should and is tolerated at the end of life), have been conceived in terms of the 'state' of the individual (usually the person who is dying). Yet, as we posit here, suffering emerges over time and across spaces as an inter-subjective assemblage, unsettling medicalised/cultural boundaries between the so-called sufferer (the one who is dying) and caring (the one who is caring for the dying person).

Notes on fieldwork

The data we draw on here was based on a programme of research lead by Alex Broom between 2011 and 2015, with the data presented below collected from 2013–2014 in Queensland, Australia, as part of a programme of research in palliative and end-of-life care. The initial period of data interviewing was conducted by Alex Broom and the second was conducted by John MacArtney, a postdoctoral researcher who was employed on the broader project. Both periods of data collection involved interviews with informal carers in palliative care settings (for example, see Broom et al., 2016). The sample included a range of relationships, including husbands, wives, long-term partners, brothers, sisters, sons, daughters, mothers, granddaughters and grandsons. The majority of the participants identified as Anglo-Australian. Almost all were caring for someone with advanced cancer.

Here, we focus on relations of care – particularly their emotions therein – and the articulation of suffering (theirs, others, both – however described and experienced). The impetus for this study in fact came from a previous study led by A. Broom in a different hospice location (see Broom, 2012; Broom & Cavenagh, 2010). That study involved spending six months immersed within a hospice, which raised considerable concerns around the moralities of the 'dying industry', as it were, and the extent to which palliative and end-of-life care was *doing things* to the dying process for different stakeholders (see Broom, 2015). One concern, which was not extrapolated on in any depth in the previous work, was how (informal) carers themselves felt during end-of-life care and the dying process, and their lived experience of suffering. This prompted a broader investigation (which we reflect on below) into the carer lifeworld, and the circulation of suffering therein.

Relational suffering and the acceptance of dying

The participants interviewed here were each at different moments in terms of their pathways to and through palliative and end-of-life care – some were in-patients, some out-patients – but each had recently, or were in the midst of, personally and interpersonally processing the fact that death was close. Yet, the notion of when a person is in fact dying is surprisingly complex, even when a person is receiving end-of-life care. 'Dying' is a contingent, conflicted and interpersonally fraught concept, mediated by medical and lay knowledges (Broom, 2015; Kellehear, 1984; Willmott, 2000; Zimmermann, 2007). Dying, as it emerged in the interviews, was highly contested, and produced, in and of itself, much angst and suffering within the carer/patient dyad or family unit. Often dying was implicit, or was 'just an idea' arrived at due to the absence of active medical intervention. Sometimes the carer would have been told that 'they were dying', and at other times nothing was said, or what was said was 'ignored'. Regardless, the transition to 'active dying' was plagued with fear and confusion from the person dying, and produced suffering for those who were caring for that person:

Kathryn: . . . so he [person dying] was very upset when he got told [that he had] three weeks [to live]. Why [had] he not received any treatment . . .? So we had to keep explaining to him. Even in the last couple of weeks, he still ask [sic], before he come to hospital 'why I'm not receiving any treatment?' He's still thinking those questions. So we have to keep explaining to him why, all the reasons, the doctor tell us why he not receive treatment because . . . it's gone too far now. Some in the liver some in the lung, so there's not much point really. [Daughter]

The above account illustrates some of the challenges for the informal carer in negotiating acknowledgement of dying, and the confusion of the person who is dying in processing the absence of active medical intervention. The majority of the carers articulated the 'living nightmare' of the (often swift) transition to the end of life, and how to manage the growing realisation for the person that they were dying, and moreover, how to manage that interpersonally:

Sarah: . . . it's really overwhelming and it's just happened so quickly. She was really good and then all of a sudden everything just went south in a big way. So it's your mind is just trying to wrap around, and everything else work and friends and everything is just out the door and you're just living this nightmare of what's happening. [Daughter]

Often the carer would be placed in a position of having to accept dying, and absorbing much of the suffering around it, whilst the person dying would either 'refuse to accept' it or 'opt out'. In this sense, much recognition of dying was filtered through, and processed by, family and carers, whose lives were 'put on hold' whilst they awaited death (this is described in greater detail below). The family and carers absorbed technical information, advice of medical futility, the dying process, and the physical deterioration likely to occur (or which was actually occurring), and attempted to manage the dying process without 'losing it':

Gavin: She is [person dying] not exactly an ostrich but sometimes she'd just prefer not to know, you know? That's why she got to a point where she didn't want any more CT scans just because she didn't want to know anymore. Because there was not really any chance that it was going to be good news, so if she could avoid it she would, and she did.

Interviewer: How was that for you?

Gavin: It was frustrating, I have to admit. She can be pretty stubborn and pig headed. And even when I know that something would benefit her, it can be frustrating when she just says 'no'. I mean, we were offered palliative radiation and she really didn't want it. [Male, Partner]

Two sites of relational suffering are reflected in the above excerpt and were articulated across the interviews. The first is the withdrawal of the person dying from acknowledgment of physical decline and the dying process. The second site is the dying person's refusal to accept palliative and supportive care due to the withdrawal of 'active treatment'. The stigma around being offered palliative care has been well- documented in existing research (Broom et al., 2013; Broom et al. 2014a; Bruera & Hui, 2010; Cherny, 2009; Miyashita et al., 2008), but this research has not focused on the relational sufferings that carers (and patients) endure as emergent from the taboos around transitions to palliative and end-of-life care. Much of the interpersonal intimacy and affection between a 'carer' and those being 'cared for' centres on the carer's support for previous medical attempts to 'try anything and everything' (often over years of intervention and care, and largely from oncologists). Acknowledgement, recognition or acceptance of dying was thus relationally fraught given the history of (collective) *fight*, *resilience* and support for *wilfulness* (cf. Ahmed, 2010, 2014). These carers and the dying person's engagement with the medical community was historically centred on the relational act (and pact) of fighting and wilfulness for life (not death) (McNamara et al., 1995; Meyer, 1995). This has created impermeable barriers to the recognition of dying, and producing suffering therein for carer and patient:

Kathy: . . . they [doctors] do keep trying to push the barrier you know, see how much you can take and it's going to make you better. But it does, it does for a while, it's [treatment has] given us eight wonderful years that we didn't think we'd have . . . But he's had enough now. But it's hard. Even today, he said '. . . we've got to start the chemo again, I haven't had chemo for a while.' So that's worrying him because he knows when he's not having chemo, the cancer's growing. So I sort of said to him '. . . you're too sick to have chemo at the moment, so we'll just wait and see'. He knows [he's dying] I'm sure, but he probably doesn't want to say anything to upset me. [Female, Partner]

Relational suffering as loss of personhood

Significantly, the carers described a fundamental change or series of 'character changes' in the person they were caring for; as though this person had become only a partial subject or even a failed self. This perceived change was often highly gendered in character, and situated within the lived experience of total pain.[1] Personhood was challenged and perceived to be lost (from the carer's perspective) during the decay and debilitation that ensued during the dying process; processes that challenged identities, role and relations between person and carer. Much of this was mourning for a previous relationship dynamic, nostalgia for previous forms of affection on the part of the carer, and the grief of being exposed to negative affect in the form of anger, resentment, desperation and hopelessness. Yet, both 'patient' and carer felt (and suffered) through, and *because of*, this. The person dying expressed their sense of 'incompleteness' to carers, and carers expressed a desire for the dying person to 'be the same as they used to be' (in the interview, to the researcher – this was never made explicit or voiced to the dying person). This is a good example of mutuality in suffering, and the co-experienced pain of the loss of the person (self and other) known and hitherto loved:

Deborah: His personality has changed, because he's in a lot of pain all the time . . . I just can't imagine how bad it must feel. So yeah he has changed, his personality has changed. He's not the happy, friendly, laughing sort of person he used to be. He's just very much focused on himself. And I've found it hard, because I said to him 'you're pushing me away. Like you're sitting there, you're looking so terribly miserable, and I'm sort of, it really impacts on me to see you looking like that.' He said 'that's how I deal with it, I just want to, leave me alone, I just want to deal with it myself, there's nothing you can do to help me' . . . but you just feel so useless. Sitting there watching that and not having that – 'what can I do?' 'nothing' – and you get pushed away. So that part is hard. Because we've been married for nearly forty years. [Wife]

Kate: The last couple of years I didn't like visiting Pop on my own, because he would tell me his disappointment in what his life had become . . . that he was ready to die. [Daughter]

Kelly: [My daughter] said 'dad's totally different to what he was.' . . . she [daughter] looks at him totally different, she said 'no, he's just a totally different person.' [Partner]

The above excerpts illustrate how this form of interpersonal struggle operates between people, and is integral to the grief of dying as a social relation and the inter-subjective character of suffering therein. The outcome of this mutual suffering in many contexts was the desire to die (patient) and the hope for death (carer), as shown below:

Kevin: It's overwhelming! It's just huge emotions, absolutely huge emotions. I want mum to – I'd love mum here, but she's so sick and I know she's going to die. But I want her to be comfortable and without pain when she dies. But I'm like 'you can't wish your mother dead.' So you've got these crazy emotions going on. [Son]

Taboo desires such as 'wish[ing] your mother dead' are expanded on further below. The above quote provides insight into an interesting dilemma for the carer in the context of mutual suffering. There is recognition of almost total loss of person and relationship, but the normative demands of informal care hold that these affective dimensions to the end of life must be supressed (Harding & Higginson, 2001; Hochschild, 1979, 1983; Mol, 2008). The qualities of intimacy, often involving touch and physical affection, exacerbated the sense of what *was* versus what *is*. Dying bodies (at least seen from the perspective of carers) recoiled when touched, further alienating the relationship from its qualities (of past) and producing a distant, partial present:

Diana: It's terrible, it's terrible . . . we're just drained, physically and emotionally . . . It's a terrible thing to say, but I'm sure other people have said it. You just wished they'd just hurry up and go because he's in agony. It's awful to see them suffer like this . . . he doesn't want us to even touch him . . . he's saying 'just leave me'. But all you can do is just hope [he goes] . . . they keep giving him morphine, sure[ly] that must soon [end his life]. [Daughter]

A key question that logically follows from what was outlined above is what drives carers to keep caring in such contexts? What keeps us caring and holds us to a relation that bears little resemblance to that relationship's history? Below, we explore some aspects of this tension, and the normative relational qualities of dying.

The moral economy of a 'good death': reciprocal, obligatory and stoical sufferings

Another key site of mutual suffering identified by the carers was the collective performance of dying well. Often articulated in terms of *mutual stoicism*, the carers were each aware of how the person dying internalised much of their pain, often performing and stating that they were 'okay with dying' and that they 'were ready'. Reflective of the 'good patient' which has been regularly discussed in the clinical literature (Proulx & Jacelon, 2004), in many cases, both carer and patient were responding to a morality of caring and dying (Tronto, 1993, 1998; Ungerson, 2006) – a set of normative constructs which offered responsibilities (acts of altruism, gift, sacrifice and so forth) but also facilitated internalised suffering:

Sophie: I guess it's good for me [that he's stoical], that's who he is, that's just his personality, but you worry about like I said how it, is he really that ok with it [dying]? I mean no-one's going to be that okay with it obviously but you know, is he hurting inside and doesn't want to tell

	anyone? Or, so I guess you worry whether he, you know, is managing and you hope that he's not keeping lots of stuff to himself and not feeling like he wants to tell anyone 'cause he doesn't want to burden them or anything like that. [Details withheld]
Joanna:	She has been [in pain] this morning without saying. She doesn't complain enough . . . So they're [palliative care staff] sort of aware of how she is. If she's said she's in pain and she hasn't told anybody, I'll make sure somebody knows . . . that's happened a couple of times. [Sister]
Ellen:	He's gone down tremendously. And see he can't eat properly now . . . he's got to have the pureed food and everything so, he's been through a heck of a lot. But he never complains, he's wonderful. [Partner]
Jennifer:	I think [death] it's going to be really soon, I don't know, I've never seen anyone pass away before. But . . . but he's saying he's in pain, he's telling us whereas before he wouldn't, he'd say he wasn't in pain, but he's [now] saying now he's in pain. And dad's not a man to complain, he's never complained but now he's saying he's in pain. [Daughter]

The participants observed the relational stoicism and 'good performances' of those they cared for and the complex feelings they had in response to such acts of dying well (Thomas et al., 2002). On the one hand, they appreciated the willingness to 'go out well' and the character that this illustrated (remembering the previous section in terms of personhood, the art of stoicism could indeed be an effective way of inserting one's *qualities* and *character* into the dying process). Quiet wilfulness (not complaining, not seeking pain relief) may fit into the moral bind of caring and dying as producing, as it were, a form of suffering.

We posit here that the performance of *coping well in death* is perhaps the most cruel of normative constructs, containing and engendering culturally-valued characteristics in our final moments (to be resilient,[2] not complain, 'put up with things', be brave and so forth). While we do not wish to reduce all acts to being 'normative', some of these cultural idealisations of personhood are ultimately implausible at the end of life (particularly in the context of cancer). For the carers, they also felt the strength of normative expectations, holding themselves to not 'feeling regret' by in turn performing the aspects of the 'good carer' to avoid the potential for shame or failure associated with 'not coping' or 'not doing enough' (Arksey & Glendinning, 2007; Thomas et al., 2002). The dynamic of sacrifice and repression of carer emotions were thus valued as components of the 'good carer':

Kathleen:	I don't want to have regrets . . . I thought, 'I'll do anything he wants so then I don't have regrets.' I said to him, 'oh I can't cope.' . . . it was tough for me but tougher for him. So I did what he wanted so I could live with myself afterwards. Does that make sense? . . . you're damned if you do and damned if you don't [as a carer]. [Partner, Female]
Bethany:	I don't think I'd ever be able to live with myself if I didn't do what I'm doing. And even today I feel like I don't do a very good job but I know that I'm doing the best that I can do in the circumstances. [Details withheld]

John: Now as far as I'm concerned, I mean, I'm committed to looking after her. You don't live with a woman for 48 years just to walk away or anything like that. So right from the word go, I've sort of said okay, this is, the four years that we've been, we're just sort of living on the basis that today is the best day we've got, so let's make the most of it. [Male, Partner]

There was in turn an institutional mediation of the moralities of caring and dying. For those who were caring for someone in the in-patient unit, there was often a sense of moral failure at allowing dying to occur in the hospital, and the failure to provide adequate care in the home:

Interviewer: How do you feel about him being here then?
Anna: Has to be, doesn't it . . .? Well I can't do it . . . it's just that I feel a bit of a rat, putting him in. But I just can't handle him at home anymore . . . It's just that deep down I feel as though I've done the wrong thing. [Female, Partner]
Lucy: I remember saying, 'I have looked after Pop for all these years. I'm going to make him go somewhere like this?' And I actually felt that I had totally failed him . . . Last Thursday night . . . he wanted to come home with me. I said, 'Pop, I can't take you home, you're too sick.' . . . And he said to me, 'do you want me to die in here?' And I said, 'Pop, this one time I just can't do what you ask of me . . . ' And after that he really didn't eat that much anymore . . . [that was it] [Granddaughter]

The institutional, palliative and hospice care context offered an additional level of relational complexity, with the intermingling of formal and informal carers within this context. As has been illustrated by scholarship in this area, there can be a level of pretence emergent from palliative and hospice care environments, whereby hospice staff construct a level of mutual acceptance of dying (dying as a natural process which one should ultimately accept) or seek to lighten the environment with humour or jovial dynamics (McNamara et al., 1995; Phillips, 1996). This is embedded in the broader wish and agenda within hospice and palliative care settings for 'good deaths', and the moral and normative qualities and responsibilities that this produces. As shown in the interviews, the desire from formal carers (nurses, doctors, social workers, psychologists and so forth) for a 'good enough death' was often juxtaposed with the realities of the person and relations, perpetuating an assumption that 'all was okay' in the dying process. This idealised view of the dying person and their dying process offered a series of moral challenges to the carers who sought an authentic, albeit stoical, subject position around the dying process:

Katrina: . . . he's raving, aggressive. The thing I found all along, there's a huge disconnect between what we see and what we know, and what medical people tell us. We're in very regularly, but the days we weren't

I'd ring up and they'd say, 'oh, he's had a great day he's fine! He's peaceful!' He's this that, and the other. And I'd be in the next day, and he'd be angry and swearing, 'get me out of here! I'm getting out of this f-ing this, that and the other.' And you'd think, 'who's crazy here?' And the nurse would come and say, 'hi [name], how are you?' and he'd say, 'alright.' 'That's good!' And what they were seeing, or they thought they were seeing, was completely wrong. And at no time did anyone in the hospital or the nursing people at [name of unit] see what we saw, and what we knew. We know the man. Don't tell us he's something else when we know him, but everyone does . . . they'd [palliative care staff] take him back, [and say] 'oh, we love him. He's our family here.' [Daughter]

The quote from Katrina captures a number of potentially important dilemmas and in turn, forms of suffering that emerge from them. And these link to the previous sections. Normative qualities of dying are performed (by carer and patient) but also perpetuated by health professionals. For example, according to Katrina, the medical staff would assure her that her father was 'peaceful' (as one is meant to be at the point of death), when his 'raving, aggressive' behaviour suggested otherwise.

'I don't even care if she dies': secrecy, loathing and hoping for death

A final aspect of relational suffering in this context is the cultural and interpersonal secrecy that operates within and across relationships, families and communities. Secrecy has important functions – particularly at the end of life and in the dying process – but it also articulates the 'back stage' realities of front stage performances. Above, we outlined the dynamics of stoicism and mutual obligation – the awareness and performance of moralities in the context of the dying process. Much suffering circulated around this dynamic for carers and patients – the co-production of a 'good death' and the moral practice of caring and dying (Burns et al., 2015; MacArtney et al., 2015b, 2017). This was both functional, but also highly problematic in other respects, for both 'carer' and 'cared for'. Yet, these stoic relations and moralities of care were often underpinned with a series of private thoughts and feelings that formed another articulation of suffering within the caring relation – those taboo, secret emotions of loathing, resentment and hoping for death (see also Olson, 2015).

Andrew: So this [caring] is a very, this is really quite hard. There's a lot of uncertainty, I guess there's a certain amount of loathing and blackness . . . [caring] it's like a form of pain or torture for every individual I think. [Son]

Julia: I think I have a lot of moments where I'm not sympathetic and a lot of times when I feel like I don't even care if she die[s]. But the reality is, I probably will be upset when she does die, but . . . [Daughter]

Katrina: . . . he's never cared who he hurt, who he let down. This is his whole life, we know him. You mean nothing to him, I mean nothing to him. . . . it's like the bare bones of the man have come out and no-one will say that . . . you look at them [parents] when it's time to show some real guts. I think it's important how you die, it's the last thing you do. For your family, for people . . . You have all these conflicting feelings. We [are] stuck in there, we didn't criticise them [parents], kept the anger hidden. But they just [parents] disgust me, the pair of them . . . I just want it to end [for him]. [Daughter]

Such secret forms of loathing, resentment or even just being 'over it', which were usually shared with no one outside the interview, were compounded by the consistent 'false alarms' that most of the carers, and certainly those in in-patient contexts, had experienced – that it was 'all over', and then the person's condition improved:

Patricia: He was pretty sick when he got here [palliative care unit]. And I think we all thought that he wouldn't make it through the next week. But they stabilised him so well that he picked up . . . it was sort of like 'well, does he have to come back home? How am I going to look after him?' That was a really anxious time . . . [Daughter]

Zoe: So you sort of, you've built up to him going and then it sort of it gets a little bit, it's a letdown, it's awful, but a letdown when he doesn't [die]. Because, I mean, you've built yourself up thinking 'this is it, this is going to be the end, it's going to happen' and then when it doesn't you think 'oh, ok, here we go again,' and you're sort of up and down up and down, it's stressful. You're sort of preparing yourself and building yourself up for this 'god he's gonna die,' and he doesn't. (Laughs) Does that sound [awful], do other people say this sort of thing? . . . Because I wonder sometimes if it's just me, am I the only person that thinks like this? [Wife]

Above we see just some of the 'taboo feelings' (as described by the participants) that exist in relation to their caring role, and in relation to the person who was dying. Clearly an articulation of suffering – sometimes over the life course, and sometimes in the specific context of dying – these feelings often centred on wanting the person to die, viewing them as weak, disappointing or lacking character, or not wanting to care for them at home any more (and thus wanting them to die). The normative framing asked these carers to be 'strong', 'stoical' and 'hopeful yet realistic' (Arksey & Glendinning, 2007; Clement, 1996; Held, 2006). The institutional environment asked them to maintain an idealised perception of the person as they were dying, ignoring negative affective dimensions including abject hopelessness, loss of personhood, melancholia, and forms of loathing and resentment (McNamara et al., 2008; Mok & Chiu, 2004). For both carer and the person dying, this encouraged a form of moral citizenship whereby the person enacts and illustrates valued characteristics. This, we posit, can function as a form of cruelty for certain patients and carers as they 'fail' to reach the standards of the (cultural) moralities of caring and dying. Their internal desires and hopes, in turn, often contrast with the cultural valorisation of the informal carer (who embarks on gift, sacrifice and stoicism within question), enhancing the impact of dying for all actors, and encouraging suffering therein.

Conclusion

In this chapter, we have sought to reassess and reconceptualise the relations of informal care for the dying, and the importance of forms of (collective and individual) suffering therein. This has challenged some core assumptions around care, caring and dying. This is set in a context whereby dominant understandings of caring relations have vastly over-emphasised the patient, as well as the erroneous split between the 'carer' and 'cared for'; and have thus positioned suffering within this binary model. This is not to say that 'patients' and 'carers' do not have specific needs or experiences. Clearly they do. Rather, we suggest that the burden of dying, the pain of mortality in all its forms (emotional, spiritual, physical, cultural) does not sit neatly within a person and, indeed, does not stay still across time and space. Suffering is shared, pain moves around families and relations, and suffering is a co-production by actors who are invested in certain practices, techniques and forms of knowledge. Dying is a collective social practice, and the atmospheres it creates (and is created by) is *achieved* by multiple actors, technologies, and discourses. Dread, horror, hope and peace are just some of the affective dimensions of dying, with individuals' experiences of dying often unsettling their normative responsibilities (as 'loving carer', as 'peaceful patient' and as 'rational doctor'). We can see suffering in these 'failures', illustrating the disciplinary character of social expectations, or concealments, of secrecy (of feelings), and of the denial of collective pain. Too often, the search for individualised solutions (to individualised models) can mean that the suffering of carers is bracketed to bereavement. In fact, carers' suffering cannot be isolated, removed and dislocated from its intersubjective origins.

We recognise that there are specific forms of suffering which people who occupy particular roles experience. As is evident in the stories provided above, the dynamics of shame, repression, and the dynamics of secrecy are *carer-specific*, but they in turn articulate relational forms of suffering, including the (mutuality of) hopelessness, powerlessness and anticipatory grief. The perceived loss of person (i.e. they are, I am, different now) was experienced concurrently. This problematic of loss of intimate connection and self/personhood reflected a relational pain and loss that was shared. Another layer of relational suffering lay in the (often dangerous) moralities of caring and dying, and the normative pressure placed on all (informal) stakeholders. This problematic was again, construed within a binary of individual responsibility (to be 'strong', 'stoical', 'resilient', illustrate 'strength of character', manage hope *and* acceptance concurrently, illustrate wilfulness and optimism in the face of death) whether aimed at 'carer' or 'cared for', was palpable in the interviews. This reflects a normativity which reproduces the binaries of caring relations, and the location of suffering within a person who is dying. Caring becomes a practice of gift-giving, sacrifice and duty as a 'good carer'.

Conversely, dying becomes an act of performing 'dignity' and 'grace', as one attempts to produce a 'good death'. The reality is these normative constructs demand that which cannot be delivered, in part because of the very nature of dying, and in part because they misconstrue the separation of roles and subject positions within the dying process. What tends to occur in the context of individualised suffering is that the dying person's suffering is recognised to an extent (albeit as an individualised process) and the carers' suffering is concealed (at least until after the patient's death, whereby the carer is offered respite in the form of a 'bereavement period'). In this context, secrecy, around emotions held by carer and patient (explored elsewhere in this book) will proliferate and create further difficulties in enacting care and coping with dying, as 'true feelings' are held back, reducing (important) forms of intimacy, exchange and recognition in the dying process. If we were, as we argue here, to position dying as together, shared, intersubjective and relational, we would go some way to better understanding what actually occurs within the dying process, and how suffering is in fact spread across, and shared between, persons.

Notes

1 The notion of total pain was developed in the palliative and hospice care movement to refer to the many different spheres of pain, including social, psychological, spiritual and physical.
2 According to Michael Unger, 'resilience' can be defined as:

> a set of behaviors over time that reflect the interactions between individuals and their environments, in particular the opportunities for personal growth that are available and accessible. . . . The likelihood that these interactions will promote well-being under adversity depends on the meaningfulness of these opportunities and the quality of the resources provided. . . . [R]esilience results from a cluster of ecological factors that predict positive human development (more that individual traits), and that the effect of an individual's capacity to cope and the resources he or she has is influenced by the nature of the challenges the individual faces.
>
> (cited in Cover, 2016, p. 353)

For an incisive analysis of 'resilience', see Cover (2016). Cover focuses on how resilience has played out in representations of queer youth.

References

Ahmed, Sara. (2010). *The Promise of Happiness*. Durham, NC: Duke University Press.
Ahmed, Sara. (2014). *Willful Subjects*. Durham, NC: Duke University Press.
Arksey, H. & Glendinning, C. (2007). Choice in the context of informal care-giving. *Health & Social Care in the Community*, 15(2), pp. 165–175.
Bailey, J. & Robertson, M. (2015). A care union in a time of austerity. *Labour & Industry*, 25(1), pp. 52–67.
Bauman, Z. (1991). *Modernity and Ambivalence*. Cambridge: Polity.

Beck, U. & Beck-Gernsheim, E. (1996) Individualization and 'precarious freedoms'. In Heelas, P., Lash, S. & Morris, P., eds., *Detraditionalization.* Oxford: Blackwell, pp. 23–48.

Berecki-Gisolf, J., Lucke, J., Hockey, R. & Dobson, A. (2008). Transitions into informal caregiving and out of paid employment of women in their 50s. *Social Science & Medicine*, 67(1), pp. 122–127.

Broom, A. (2012). On euthanasia, resistance and redemption: The moralities and politics of a hospice. *Qualitative Health Research*, 22(2), pp. 226–237.

Broom, A. (2015). *Dying: A Social Perspective on the End of Life*. London and New York: Routledge.

Broom, A. & Cavenagh, J. (2010). Moralities, masculinities and caring for the dying: An exploration of experiences of living and dying in a hospice. *Social Science and Medicine*, 71(5), pp. 869–876.

Broom, A. & Kirby, E. (2013). The end of life and the family: Hospice patients' views on dying as relational. *Sociology of Health and Illness*, 35(4), pp. 499–513.

Broom, A., Kirby, E., Good, P. & Lwin, Z. (2015a). Nursing futility, managing medicine: Nurses' perspectives on the transition from life-prolonging to palliative care. *Health*. http://journals.sagepub.com/doi/abs/10.1177/1363459315595845 (accessed 1/10/16).

Broom, A., Kirby, E., Adams, J. & Refshuage, K. (2015b). On illegitimacy, suffering and recognition: A diary study of women living with chronic pain. *Sociology*, 49(4), pp. 712–731.

Broom, A. Kirby, E., Kenny, K., MacArtney, J. & Good, P. (2016). Moral ambivalence and informal care for the dying. *The Sociological Review*, 64(4), pp. 987–1004.

Broom, A., Kirby, E., Good, P., Wootton, J. & Adams, J. (2013). The art of letting go: Referral to palliative care and its discontents. *Social Science and Medicine*, 78, pp. 9–16.

Broom, A., Kirby, E., Good, P., Wootton, J. & Adams, J. (2014a). The troubles of telling: Managing communication about the end of life. *Qualitative Health Research*, 24(2), pp. 151–162.

Broom, A., Kirby, E., Good, P., Wootton, J., Hardy, J. & Yates, P. (2014b). Negotiating futility, managing emotions: Nursing the transition to palliative care. *Qualitative Health Research*, 25(3), pp. 299–309.

Bruera, E. & Hui, D. (2010). Integrating supportive and palliative care in the trajectory of cancer: Establishing goals and models of care. *Journal of Clinical Oncology*, 28(25), pp. 4013–4017.

Bubeck, Diemut. 1995. *Care, Gender, and Justice*. Oxford: Clarendon Press.

Burns, E. J., Quinn, S. J., Abernethy, A. P. & Currow, D. C. (2015). Caregiver expectations: Predictors of a worse than expected caregiving experience at the end of life. *Journal of Pain and Symptom Management*, 50(4), pp. 453–461.

Chattoo, S. & Ahmad, W. I. U. (2008). The moral economy of selfhood and caring. *Sociology of Health & Illness*, 30(4), pp. 550–564.

Cherny, N. (2009). Stigma associated with 'palliative care'. *Cancer*, 115(9), pp. 1808–1812.

Clement, G. (1996). *Care, Autonomy, and Justice*. Boulder, CO: Westview Press.

Cover, R. (2016). Resilience. In Rodriguez, N., Martino, W., Ingrey, J. & Brockenbrough, E., eds., *Critical Concepts in Queer Studies and Education: An International Guide for the Twenty-First Century*. New York: Palgrave Macmillan, pp. 351–360.

Currow, D. C., Burns, C., Agar, M., Phillips, J., McCaffrey, N. & Abernethy, A. P. (2011). Palliative caregivers who would not take on the caring role again. *Journal of Pain and Symptom Management*, 41(4), pp. 661–672.

Doka, K. J., ed. (2002). *Disenfranchised Grief: New Directions, Challenges, and Strategies for Practice*. Champaign, IL: Research Press.

Fisher, B. & Tronto, J. (1990). Toward a feminist theory of care. In Abel, E. and Nelson, M., eds., *Circles of Care*. Albany, NY: State University of New York Press, pp. 35–62.

Harding, R. & Higginson, I. (2001). Working with ambivalence: Informal caregivers of patients at the end of life. *Supportive Care in Cancer*, 9(8), pp. 642–645.

Held, V. (2006). *The Ethics of Care*. Oxford, New York: Oxford University Press.

Hochschild, A. R. (1979). Emotion work, feeling rules, and social structure. *American Journal of Sociology*, 85(3), pp. 551–575.

Hochschild, A. (1983). *The Managed Heart*. Berkeley, CA: University of California Press.

Kellehear, A. (1984). Are we a death denying society? A sociological review. *Social Science and Medicine*, 18(9), pp. 713–723.

Kittay, E. (1999). *Love's Labor: Essays on Women, Equality, and Dependency*. New York: Routledge.

MacArtney, J., Broom, A., Kirby, E., Good, P. & Wootton, J. (2017). The liminal and the parallax: Living and dying at the end of life. *Qualitative Health Research*, 27(5), pp. 623–633. http://journals.sagepub.com/doi/pdf/10.1177/1049732315618938.

MacArtney, J. I., Broom, A., Kirby, E., Good, P., Wootton, J., Yates, P. M. & Adams, J. (2015a). On resilience and acceptance in the transition to palliative care at the end of life. *Health*, 19(3), pp. 263–279.

MacArtney, J., Broom, A., Kirby, E., Good, P., Wootton, J. & Adams, J. (2015b). Locating care at the end of life: Burden, vulnerability, and the practical accomplishment of dying. *Sociology of Health and Illness*, 38(3), pp. 479–492. DOI: 10.1111/1467-9566.12375

McNamara, B., Waddell, C. & Colvin, M. (1995). Threats to the good death: The cultural context of stress and coping among hospice nurses. *Sociology of Health & Illness*, 17(2), pp. 222–241.

Meyer, M. (1995). Dignity, death and modern virtue. *American Philosophical Quarterly*, 32, pp. 45–56.

Miyashita, M., Hirai, K., Morita, T., Sanjo, M. & Uchitomi, Y. (2008). Barriers to referral to inpatient palliative care units in Japan: A qualitative survey with content analysis. *Support Care Cancer*, 16(3), pp. 217–222.

Mok, E. & Chiu, P. C. (2004). Nurse–patient relationships in palliative care. *Journal of Advanced Nursing*, 48(5), pp. 475–483.

Mol, A. (2008). *The Logic of Care*. London and New York: Routledge.

Olson, R. (2015). When they don't die: Prognosis ambiguity, role conflict and emotion work in cancer caregiving. *Journal of Sociology*, 51(4), pp. 857–871.

Phillips, S. (1996). Labouring the emotions: Expanding the remit of nursing work? *Journal of Advanced Nursing*, 24(1), pp. 139–143.

Proulx, K. & Jacelon, C. (2004). Dying with dignity: The good patient versus the good death. *American Journal of Hospice and Palliative Care*, 21(2), pp. 116–120.

Thomas C., Morris, S. M. & Harman, J. C. (2002). Companions through cancer. *Social Science & Medicine*, 54(4), pp. 529–544.

Tronto, J. (1993). *Moral Boundaries: A Political Argument for an Ethic of Care*. New York: Routledge.

Tronto, J. (1998). An ethic of care. *Generations*, 22(3), pp. 15–20.

Twigg J. & Atkin, K. (1994). *Carers Perceived*. Buckingham: Open University Press.

Ungerson, C. (2006). Care, work and feeling. *The Sociological Review*, 53(s2), pp. 188–203.

West, R. (2002). The right to care. In Kittay, E.F. & Feder, E., eds., *The Subject of Care: Feminist Perspectives on Dependency*. Lanham, MD: Rowman and Littlefield.

Willmott, H. (2000). Death. So what? Sociology, sequestration and emancipation. *The Sociological Review*, 48(4), pp. 649–665.

Zimmermann, C. (2007). Death denial: Obstacle or instrument for palliative care? An analysis of clinical literature. *Sociology of Health & Illness*, 29(2), pp. 297–314.

Part 2

Suffering, the lived body and mobility

3 The practice of secrecy as a moral economy of care
Affect, fragility and intergenerational suffering

Introduction

In this chapter, we argue that hauntings (Derrida, 1994; Gordon, 2008) offer a useful conceptual way of capturing the presence of affect, which is often felt and lived as suffering. Our exploration of suffering as an affective assemblage of human bodies, matter and things, discourses, practices and performances is focused on the analysis of intergenerational suffering caused by historical violence, and of family secrecy about the biological relatedness of children fathered by enemy soldiers. Regardless of how these children were conceived, their mothers would give a birth to an 'open secret'.[1] Our analysis here is focused on people born to Indisch (Indonesian-Dutch) mothers and Japanese fathers during the Japanese occupation of the Dutch East Indies, from 1942 to 1945. Here, the child's body becomes evidence of sexual and racial transgression. The ethnographic material we analyse urges us to problematise the understanding of the human body as a singular, bounded entity, and the effect of intergenerational distress as located solely in the singular bodies of the victims of historical violence. Our focus is on how the effects of historical violence and the concealment of knowledge about biological relatedness to former wartime enemies are shaped, constituted, contested and sustained as affective assemblages. Thus, our particular focus is on *what assemblages do* (Deleuze & Guattari, 1987, p. 257), and our analysis calls for the reconsideration of the value of current logics of trauma, including Post-Traumatic Stress Disorder. We argue that understanding intergenerational suffering goes beyond individual psychopathology.

The predominant psychological paradigm stresses that children of the survivors of different forms of historical violence – including the Holocaust, the Second World War, the Vietnam War, invaded indigenous peoples, and repressive regimes – develop psychological trauma symptoms (Danieli, 2010). Since the 1980s, psychological trauma symptoms have been included in the American Psychiatric Association's Diagnostic and Statistical Manual of Mental Disorders (DSM-III) (the third edition in 1980 and subsequent editions) under the name 'Post-Traumatic Stress Disorder' (hereafter referred to as 'PTSD'). Following this paradigm, legacies of violence have been defined as a 'conspiracy of silence' between survivors and society, and have been experienced as a sense of acute pain, haplessness and anger (Danieli, 2010, p. xv).

Since the first formulation of the definition of PTSD in the 1980s, it has been widely accepted that war causes trauma for both victims and perpetrators. Anthropologists Didier Fassin and Richard Rechtman (2009) have cogently argued: 'Trauma has become a major signifier of our age. It is our normal means of relating present suffering to past violence' (ibid., p. xi).[2]

Over the last several decades, intergenerational transmission of trauma has been studied across a number of different fields such as psychoanalysis (e.g. Abraham & Torok, 1994; Davoine and Gaudilliere, 2004), memory studies (e.g. Hirsch, 2008; Hirsch & Smith, 2002; Hoffman, 2010), the interdisciplinary fields of critical psychology, cultural and gender studies (Blackman, 2012; Cho, 2008; Dragojlovic, 2011, 2014, 2015a, b; Walkerdine, 2010), anthropology (Argenti & Schramm, 2010; Crapanzano, 2011; Feuchtwang, 2011; Kidron, 2009, 2012) and neurobiology and epigenetics (Yehuda, 2006). The universality of PTSD diagnostics has been criticised by anthropologists as being Eurocentric, imposing Western understandings of health and healing throughout the world, rather than attending to the multitude of ways in which responses to violence and suffering might differ across cultures (Argenti and Schramm, 2012; Eyerman, 2002; Fassin & Rechtman, 2009; Kidron, 2012). Anthropologist Carol Kidron (2009), who has analysed Holocaust survivors, offers a trenched critique of the PTSD paradigm and 'talk therapy' as universal models for healing.[3] In addition to problematising the PTSD paradigm, the field of transcultural psychiatry made an important contribution to rethinking the intergenerational impact of historical violence by introducing the concept of historical trauma, being 'the long-term impact of colonization, cultural suppression, and historical oppression of many Indigenous peoples' (Kirmayer et al., 2014, p. 300). This conceptualisation of historical trauma offers a more complex understanding of historical violence than traditional accounts that use the PTSD framework, as it merges understandings of historical oppression with psychological experiences of trauma (ibid.).

This chapter builds on and diverges from the previous scholarship in three important ways. First, aside from a few exceptions (Blackman 2012; Cho, 2008; Dragojlovic, 2015a, b; To, 2015), the scholarship on intergenerational transmission of trauma and distress has been predominantly focused on individual humans and their psychological states. Here, instead, we are interested in analysing emotional distress as an affective assemblage of human and non-human processes (Blackman, 2012) in order to problematise the dichotomy of the ill and the healthy body, and to focus on processes of becoming, including the potential for self-transformation.

Second, we offer a detailed ethnographic account of the intergenerational practice of secrecy as an affective *moral economy of caring* wherein 'emotions do things' (Ahmed, 2004, p. 119), which is reinforced by heteronormativity and the effects of structural racism that reverberate across generations. Unlike Danieli's 'conspiracy of silence' (2010, p. xv), wherein trauma is perceived to reside within a singular psychological subject, we posit that the practice of secrecy is an affective assemblage constituent of human bodies, matter, things, discourses, practices and performances, and is a modality of intergenerational haunting.

Third, we argue that affective connections to historical violence should not be seen as either 'cultural' or 'psychological' (including PTSD and related anxiety disorders). This is because such arguments are embedded in a problematic separation between the mind and the body, nature and culture. Rather, we suggest that the multifaceted forms of historical violence, structural racism, gendered inequalities and related marginalisation alert us to the fragility of the embodied individual and our collective selves. Thus, building on queer, feminist and critical race scholarship (Ahmed, 2010; Blackman, 2015; Cvetkovich, 2012; Halberstam, 2011; Love, 2007), we explore the potentially productive and transformative possibilities of negative feelings.

Here, through an ethnographic lens, we explore how affectivity operates through and across the binary oppositions of cognitive and affective, and intentional and non-intentional (see also Blackman, 2012; Leys, 2011; Navaro-Yashin, 2012), individual and collective. Furthermore, as in the rest of the book, we offer a critique of the banishment of the subject from affect studies, and argue that attention must be paid to how affectivity is qualified and given meaning by the subject (see also Blackman, 2012; Dragojlovic 2015b; Navaro-Yashin, 2012). Lisa Blackman's (2012, p. 1) argument that 'rather than talk about bodies, we might instead talk of brain-body-world entanglements' is particularly pertinent when engaging with intergenerational experiences of distress in order to approach the lived body beyond the singular psychological subject and towards a more intersubjective and intercorporeal understanding (see also Csordas, 2008). Such an approach allows us to unsettle the dichotomies of human and non-human (matter and things), and the now versus historic experience, and to think about intergenerational suffering as both collective and individual.

Research methods

This chapter forms part of a larger, ongoing anthropological research project on Indisch memory and genealogy work that Dragojlovic began in 2009. As part of this anthropological research, Dragojlovic conducted open-ended, semi-structured interviews with 189 individuals, and participated in various social and family events. At the beginning, participants were solicited formally through community networks and social media platforms such as Facebook. Participation then grew through informal solicitations to further potential participants at social gatherings and community events. By also closely following the dynamics within 23 Indisch families over a period of five years, Dragojlovic was able to develop longitudinal and in-depth insights that would have been unachievable if her research had been based solely on structured, formal interviews. Throughout this project, she relied on various ethnographic techniques including recording genealogies, examining past and present family relationships. Dragojlovic also critically observed current social and cultural engagements.

The interlocutors narrated their family histories in the form of semi-structured interviews and informal conversations at family gatherings or Indisch cultural activities. An integral part of each semi-structured interview was the inquiry into the interlocutors' possession of legal documents such as birth certificates, residency permits and proofs of citizenship, and visual material such as family photographs and drawings related to the family's history as selected by the inter-locutors. Additionally, the interlocutors drew family trees; a task which in most cases proved to be a difficult and, on occasion, daunting task, revealing stories of past suffering, bitterness, suspicion and betrayal during the Second World War, the Indonesian struggle for independence, and the subsequent decolonisation (see also Dragojlovic, 2011). In her previous work, Dragojlovic explored how Indisch people's intergenerational 'incorporated body memory' (Leys, 2013) grapples with memories of places left by their ancestors in the colonial Dutch East Indies as a result of wars, imprisonment and torture (see Dragojlovic, 2011, 2014, 2015a, 2016). Dragojlovic approaches memories not only as constructed but as being sediment in the bodies, wherein bodies are carriers of memory, which is often unconsciously incorporated (Connerton, 1989).

In what follows, we offer a brief interlude into Indisch and Indisch-Japanese history, which forms an integral part of the affective assemblages of intergenera-tional suffering we discuss in this chapter. This interlude aims to help the reader situate other elements of the assemblage and their linkages that are analysed later in this chapter. It is important to stress that the scholarly literature reviewed here was almost without exception an important part of the interlocutors' libraries, as affective matter – that is, matter that is capable of discharging energy and creating an intense atmosphere of close proximity to the events and places of the Dutch East Indies.[4]

Indisch and Indisch-Japanese people: a brief historical interlude

The formation of Indisch cultures began in the colonial Dutch East Indies, which is the present day Indonesia (Bosma & Raben, 2008). From the early seventeenth century onwards, European (mainly Dutch) men took Indonesian women as their companions, either as legitimate wives or as so-called *nyai* (housekeepers/bed partners), which resulted in a large Indo-European population. Over the centuries, this practice was normalised (Locher-Scholten, 1995; Taylor, 1983) and interra-cial intimacies were accepted as long as they followed prescribed gender, race and class patterns. Indisch people and communities in the Dutch East Indies occupied an ambivalent space – on the one hand, they were granted privileges reserved for Europeans, but on the other, they were able to move between European and Indo-nesian worlds (Stoler, 2002). While the population of the Dutch East Indies was divided into three seemingly clear categories – Europeans (*Europeanen*), natives (*Inlanders*) and Foreign Asians (*Vreemde Oosterlingen*) – each of these categories was multi-layered, with the category of 'Europeans' being particularly so (Stoler, 2002). Before the ethical policy (*ethische politiek*) was enunciated in 1900, the Europeans were divided into two main categories – permanent and temporary res-idents, with the permanent residents (*Blijvers*) including both people of multira-cial descent and 'pure' whites (*Blanda totok*). Indo-Europeans (*Indo-Europeanen*) were able to acquire the juridical status of 'European' only after their fathers were formally recognised as such (Pattynama, 2000).

The Japanese occupation of the Dutch East Indies (1942–1945) constituted the beginning of the end of the Dutch East Indies. The Japanese introduced new racial classifications wherein Indo-Europeans/'Eurasians' came to be classified as 'Asians' rather than 'Europeans'. While the majority of the European population was interned in prison camps, those of Eurasian origin were given the opportunity to avoid being sent to the prison camps if they succeeded in proving a desirable degree of Indonesian background. Approximately 100,000 Dutch and Eurasian individuals were interned, while approximately 220,000 Eurasians were able to avoid the Japanese prison camps (de Jong, 2002). Living conditions were especially harsh for women and children at this time, regardless of whether they were living within or outside the camps.

It is important to stress here that, prior to the Second World War, the Dutch colonial notion of superiority often casted images of Japanese people as inferior; as 'intrusive, repulsive and subhuman, as people with an evil nature' (Buchheim, 2007, p. 268). Around 100,000 women served as so-called 'comfort women', being forced into prostitution during the Pacific War in China and Southeast Asia (Buchheim, 2007, p. 261). These 'comfort women' (*ianfu*, jap.; a euphemism for women forced into prostitution; see Ezawa, 2015, p. 481) were mobilised as a 'military supply'; Japanese Army and Navy planners generally determined to have one comfort woman available per 40 soldiers at the frontline (Buchheim, 2007, p. 261). During this period, an unknown number of Indisch women had consensual intimate encounters with Japanese soldiers and servicemen. After the end of the Second World War (1945) and Indonesian independence (internationally recognised in 1949), Indisch people, being Dutch citizens, moved from Indonesia to the Netherlands, Australia, the United States and Canada. Over time, they came to be characterised as a 'model minority'[5] within these countries. Within the broader network of Indisch communities, Indisch-Japanese people occupy an ambivalent space. Being fathered by enemy soldiers during the Second World War, they are an embodiment of Indisch women's intimate relationships with the enemy, but also a reminder of the end of the Dutch colonial empire, which was brought down by a series of events that began with the Japanese occupation. Such paradoxical sentiments are reflected in Indisch-Japanese people's ambiguous feelings about Indisch communities and networks, which range from a sense of 'unfair marginalisation', to concealment of one's Japanese genealogy in Indisch circles, to a complete lack of interest in, or rejection of, Indisch events.

Secrecy as a moral economy of care

> What if the truth is not so much a secret as a *public secret*, as is the case with the most important knowledge, *knowing what not to know*'
>
> (Taussig, 1999, p. 51)

Documented narratives about the circumstances under which Indisch women engaged in intimate relationships with Japanese men during the Japanese occupation describe the relationships as ranging from romantic to casual; from relationships strategically engaged in as a protection strategy during the hardships of the war, to romanticised representations of long-term loving relationships. Very occasionally, some narratives hint at the possibility of the Japanese man having coerced the Indisch woman into the relationship (Buchheim, 2007; Ezawa, 2015). Whatever their origins or nature, though, while these relationships may have been acceptable and tolerated during the occupation, this changed once the war ended. After the war, knowledge about such relationships became (in most cases) a carefully guarded family secret (see also Ezawa, 2015). Evelin Buchheim (2007, p. 272) has noted that long-term relationships between Japanese men and Indisch women were discouraged by the Japanese military, primarily because of the fear of the Indisch women engaging in espionage and bribery. As a result, many ongoing relationships between Japanese men and Indisch women were couched in secrecy, occurring exclusively within the private sphere.

Regardless of the kind of intimate encounters Indisch women had with Japanese men during the war, the presence of Indisch-Japanese children following the end of the occupation presented many difficulties. Some of the Indisch women who had intimate relations with Japanese men had had husbands before the war. Where these men survived the Japanese internment camps, this created issues when they returned home after the war. On the other hand, many Indisch women lost family members, including husbands, in the Japanese camps. Those women whose husbands were interned in the camps often claimed that the children they gave birth to shortly after their husbands went to war or were interned were conceived within their regular marital relationships, rather than through relations with Japanese men. Some family members, friends or acquaintances knew all too well that such claims were made under pressure to conceal knowledge about the biological fathers of their children. Under such difficult circumstances, some children were given to orphanages, while others were adopted by relatives and presented as children found or born out of legitimate Indisch–Indisch marital unions just after the commencement of the, war. Aside from some rare cases, the biological relatedness of Indisch-Japanese children was carefully guarded throughout these children's lives. Many such children fathered by Japanese men had no knowledge about their biological fathers until they entered middle age. Some Indisch-Japanese people grew up believing that their mother's husband, and often biological father of the other siblings, was their biological father, too. Others were made to believe that their biological father died during the war and that their mothers married again later on. Only a small minority knew all their life that their father was a Japanese man. As in many other war situations, women's sexuality was not only perceived as a matter of personal choice but as a sign of national and/or ethnic honour, and women's reproductive capacities were regarded as a national resource (Ericsson & Simonsen, 2005). As has been seen in different post-war contexts, women who had transgressed normative expectations and had intimate relationships and/or bore children out of consensual intimate relationships with the enemy faced many forms of retribution (ibid.).

Dragojlovic met all of her Indisch-Japanese interlocutors at a point in their lives when they were already part of Indisch-Japanese social networks and when they were (as many described it) 'working on the past'. Without exception, her interlocutors stressed that they had grown up in an atmosphere of typical Indisch silence (Indisch *zwijgen*), which many felt had generated a very distinct sense of malaise that ran deeply but was often difficult to articulate verbally. Their parents' difficult pasts pervaded their own present, creating an atmosphere in which past sufferings were simultaneously elusive and omnipresent, and frequently produced a sense of othering among the children as they struggled to navigate through their everyday lives. While the notion of secrets and hidden knowledge within Indisch families is frequently referred to as 'typically Indisch', the common understanding is that what has been silenced or only whispered about are detailed particularities about past suffering caused by war, sexual coercion and violence, and a general sense of bitterness caused by a sense of betrayal by friends, relatives and the postcolonial Dutch state. Such circumstances produced what we refer to as a 'practice of secrecy'. In the detailed ethnographic accounts that follow, we demonstrate how the practice of secrecy can be defined as an element of the affective assemblage constituted by irregular verbal and non-verbal articulation about the past, mediated by divergent forms of concealment and revelation.

For Dragojlovic's interlocutors, the practice of secrecy was an attempt to 'leave the past behind' troubled by feelings of suffering and their visceral experiences of anger, discontent and depression. Secrecy, as a foundational sociological principle (Simmel, 1906), is an important aspect that builds and sustains relationships and communities.[6] Secrets are paradoxical in themselves as they come into existence when extracted into narrative (Derrida, 2001) and are manifested through traces that represent something that is inaccessible or hard to comprehend (Butler, 2005; Derrida, 2001). Thus, secrets are discursive and performative, but also material and affective. As the ethnographic material demonstrates, in this case, the practice of secrecy emanates as an affective, *moral economy of caring*, and is reinforced by heteronormativity and the effects of structural racism that reverberates across generations. In other words, we explore how complex sets of moralities surrounding female propriety during the war, normative expectations of family life (namely, nuclear families consisting of biological parents and their children), and forms of obligation (wherein parents or adults in general care for children regardless of who their biological fathers might be) are enmeshed in practices of care. We explore how tensions between moral expectations to care for children (in this case fathered by enemy soldiers) and personal psychological injury caused by the wartime enemy leads biological (mothers) and social (step-fathers) parents to be complicit in the perpetuation of affective distress. Yet, as the ethnographic material discussed here demonstrates, the moral economy of caring is not limited to the nuclear family; instead, the extended family and the society as a whole are implicit in the intergenerational suffering assemblages. Thus, we explore how the practices of secrecy as a moral economy of caring are crucial elements of the affective assemblages of intergenerational suffering and, based on the ethnographic material presented here, cannot be limited to the individual psychopathology.

The narratives that follow were told to Dragojlovic as part of personal reflections by her interlocutors on the discovery of the biological make-up of their parents; a discovery which almost without exception brought about intensified affective states that disrupted her interlocutors' everyday lives, necessitating powerful reconfigurations of the self. These reconfigurations ranged from cognitive awareness, critical reflection and public articulation about historical trauma, to medical diagnostics of 'burnout', 'secondary PTSD' and 'depression', intensifying the experiences of intergenerational suffering. In what follows, Dragojlovic offers two lengthy narratives in order to ethnographically explore what *affective assemblages of suffering do*, by exploring how affective intensities are registered in the body, the affective intensities of matter and things, and how these are subjectively given meaning. The two narratives poignantly illustrate the multifaceted aspects of care, demonstrating how moral economy of caring is embedded in affective forces of structural racism and gender inequalities.

Miranda: I was at the *Pasar Malam* [an annual Eurasian festival established in 1959] in 2003, casually browsing through the program, when I spotted an announcement for a talk by Indisch-Japanese children, and something in me erupted. I began to shake and felt as if the ground was disappearing under my feet; I was struggling to breathe and I thought I was having a heart attack. Somebody from the crowd helped me to sit down, brought me something to drink, and called over a paramedic. I soon calmed down and remembered being told that I was having a panic attack, and being asked whether I'd seen something upsetting. I then remembered the Indisch-Japanese talk. In the meantime, a friend with whom I had come to the Pasar joined me, and I told her that I really wanted to go to the talk. We went together and . . . ehhh . . . that was something! It was like I was in a trance . . . everything they were saying was *so* painful. There was this pain in me and they were talking to that pain which became so big, bigger than me and all the people in that large venue . . . It is hard to explain. I was so overwhelmed. Afterwards, my friend asked if I wanted to talk to her and, trying to comfort me, she said, 'But you have known for years already'. I was like, 'What do you mean? I have known what?' I was getting upset again and she said, 'about your Japanese father, you told me years ago before we went to the university.'

And of course I remembered it then; I was in my early 20s, rummaging through stuff in the attic, when I discovered my dad's diary to find out that he was in Thailand from 1943 and only reunited with my mom in 1948 – and I was born in 1945. That was a terrible, terrible shock! I rushed to my mom to ask her about it, but she became mad with me, calling me an 'ungrateful Japanese bastard', saying that she was sick of having to care for me, that caring for me only brought her troubles. She told me to 'get lost' as I had caused her enough grief already. When I left our country town, it was after an argument which

was nothing out of the ordinary in my family, but I completely, completely erased the memory of finding out about my Japanese father
and telling my friend about it! I love my mother. I know she suffered.
I cared for her and, because of that, I wanted to forget.

I spent the better part of my life avoiding all things Indisch and
Japanese, but after that day at the Pasar, things changed. I already
had a very stressful situation at work and with the shock of finding
out – *again!* – about my Japanese roots, I collapsed. All energy was
gone from my body, just like that. I was tested for all sorts of medical conditions and finally diagnosed with burnout. I realised I had
to take it easy and started doing integrative psychotherapy. In the
process, I slowly began to read about Japan and its culture. Along
the way, I realised I stopped hating it and, well, accepted this inheritance, really. Two of my children are fine with it, but my youngest
daughter does not want to know anything about being Indisch or
Japanese. She just wants to be Dutch. Being so blond and white, it's
easy for her not to have to think about her Asian heritage. [Miranda,
an Indisch-Japanese woman]

Miranda's narrative poignantly illuminates the fluidity that can exist between
what is cognitively known (the truth about her father being Japanese) and
unknown (the rediscovery of this truth at the Pasar Malam), suggesting how the
practice of secrecy can exist within a continuum of cognitive and affective, visible and invisible. The pain Miranda experiences while learning about the talk is
at first inexplicable, but nonetheless located in the narrative of others, the images
they were presenting and the atmosphere of the event, which was dedicated to
Indisch history. The sense of pain that at first she cannot explain connects to the
pain emanating from the event. Thus, the pain and distress she experiences cannot
be located solely in an individual 'I'. Instead, bodies (hers/others) show a capacity 'to affect and be affected' (Massumi, 2002, p. 61); yet, at the same time, such
capacity needs to be situated within specific historical contingencies.

Similarly, Miranda's narrative illustrates how affectivity is both intentional
(going to the event) and non-intentional (being taken over by emotions and
collapsing). Equally fluid is the notion of the healthy and the ill human body –
Miranda was 'healthy' prior to her arrival at the event, but became 'ill' when
suffering the anxiety attack, then returned to 'healthy' again once the source of
her anxiety was located. In this way, Miranda's narrative sheds light on how the
affective economy of care is multidimensional, destabilising the idea that care for
others produces harmonious relations.

Kim: I always knew that I was born in Bandung in Java in 1944. Ineke, my
mom [an Indisch woman] and Tom, my dad [an Indisch man] were great
parents; I had no trouble with them. They were great parents. I didn't feel
like they did not treat me like their own son; yes, I was the eldest and took
care of my younger siblings, but that was the case in big families back

then. There were some strange things about my travel papers when I was young. We travelled around different countries a lot and there were always only problems with mine. I thought that was because I was the only one who was born in the Dutch East Indies. I never asked why.

When we lived in Indonesia in the 1950s, where my dad had a very nice upper-middle class job at an international company, local kids shouted 'Japanese, Japanese' at me because I had a Japanese face, but I never asked my parents about it. I had this gut feeling that I was somehow irrevocably different, so I was upset by the kids, but you know, could not ask anything. Talking about family history in Indisch families is not something you do. Of course, I knew that something was not the way it should be . . . Look at these two [showing photograph of his younger siblings], true light skinned Indisch kids, and see me . . . Haha . . . anyhow . . . We were a happy family; we enjoyed the luxuries of upper-middle class families and my parents were a happy, very nice couple.

When I was about 15, I saw the papers about my adoption. They were not given to me; I found them in the desk of my father. For years, I had known something was different about me, but I was also afraid of finding out what it was. But then I saw it, and naaa yaaaaa . . . life goes on. Indisch families are complicated. I didn't talk about it with my parents, but when I was about to enter university I needed a copy of my birth certificate and it was then that my father told me that I was adopted. My father told me that they had found me in an orphanage in Bandung [Java] and, as Ineke had lost her own child prior to that, she wanted to adopt an orphan. I did not know then that it was not the complete story. I never talked about adoption with my parents; I was very close to my mother but we never talked about it. They cared for me and even though I really wanted to know more, I didn't ask them. I cared for them and did not want to upset them or make them unhappy. It was enough that they cared for me.

One day, when I was 48, my father (who had serious heart problems at the time) asked me if I could come to his house because he wanted to tell me something before he died. I came to his house and he said, 'Would you like to know who your mother is?' And I was like, 'My mother???' And then he told me that my mother was actually my aunt, one of his cousins. I do not know how (he was very uncomfortable saying this), but she got pregnant by a Japanese soldier. That was such a *big shock* for me because she was living here in the *Javaplein* [suburb in close proximity where he was living], and I've been living here in Amsterdam since I was 20. Of course, I had known her, but just as one of my aunties . . . just as an aunt in Amsterdam. And my dad said to me, 'I do not know what happened during those years, but you should talk to Anneke, the oldest sister of your biological mother.' So I contacted Anneke, whom I had also known for years, and she told me, 'my younger sister was pregnant with you and this was a big shame in the family because she was already married. Her husband was in the Japanese camp and she already had a child. She did not want to have you as a child and then it was decided within the family that you should be adopted within the family, and Ineke, who had just lost her child, decided to take you.' Anneke also told me that I was born on 26 November, which was different from my papers. Then, of course, I wanted to talk to my biological mother and ask her about my biological father, but I was *totally shocked*! It took me a month to realise what had happened, and then I received a phone call from Anneke telling me that my biological mother had died. I never had a chance to talk to her. I got *very, very sick* soon after this. I developed heart problems and became seriously depressed. It was hard – almost impossible – to talk to anyone. I stopped working. I didn't care about anything. I spent months just being in my room, barely eating . . . My wife and my son tried to help me. They took me to seek medical help but I lost my voice, my energy. I was alive, but I felt as if life had left me. I was a zombie. Haha . . . na yaaa . . . I understand now that my biological mother abandoned me because she cared about me, because she wanted to protect me. . . . We all cared about each other. We all suffered . . . [Kim, Indisch-Japanese man]

Kim's narrative draws our attention to the multifaceted, affective entanglements of care and suffering and is especially revealing about multifaceted aspects of secrecy and caring relations. We can see in both Miranda's and Kim's narratives, how the moral *economy of caring* operates as affective dynamics informed by gendered and racialised moralities, normative obligations of duty, and loyalty that necessitates an *ongoing self-contestation of the self*. The practice of secrecy that surrounds biological relatedness to the enemy (a Japanese man) is interwoven with gender normativity and the policing of female sexuality in times of war, wherein the secrecy itself becomes a moral economy of care. In the interlocutors' narratives, it was primarily extended family members of the mother who, following the end of the Japanese occupation, made the decision as to how to take care of the child or children fathered by Japanese soldiers. In this context, caring relations are embedded in power relations of gender normativity and racial hierarchies, the latter valuing white, European higher than Asian, especially as regards Japanese men, who were also the war enemies at the time.

Moral values are central to the understanding of care arrangements as well as family, biological and social reproduction flowing from Indisch-Japanese intimate relations. Narratives about care for Indisch-Japanese children in the postwar years were promoted as necessary safety measures for the children by their mothers and by her extended network of kin relations. Yet, the practice and relations of care should not be seen as one-dimensional – parents and adult relatives simply caring for children – nor should the caring relationships of adults towards children be seen as always having the best intentions. Similarly, we should not expect caring intentions to always have positive outcomes. Instead, it is important to problematise the normalisation of care and caring relations and pay more attention to the power relations that exist in these interactions. These interactions are embedded in gender normativity and racial hierarchies of biological and social reproduction becoming that (in this case) include affective intensities of intergenerational suffering.

Rather than being approached as one directional, the relationship of care between caregivers (parents) and care receivers (children) needs to be approached as multidirectional (see also Thelen, 2015). As we argue throughout this book, attention must be paid to the tensions and power relations that exist within relations of care, rather than for it to be presumed that caring intentions and the relations they produce are a stabilising force. Furthermore, any nuanced analysis of relations of care needs to be informed by moral values that underline the notion of care in a given context, and to examine the tensions and ruptures that might shift notions of what 'good' care might stand for. In the Indisch–Japanese case, practices of care were embedded in practices of secrecy and the disguise of children's biological fathers, both of which practices shaped a multifaceted moral economy of care, rooted in care for social order, gender normativity and racial purity. In this moral economy of *care as secrecy*, the biological relatedness is rendered unimportant. Yet at the same time, it is this very biological relatedness that is the source of tension and discontent.

The practice of secrecy and the feeling body

In this section, we pay close attention to how intergenerational and intercorporeal experiences of intergenerational suffering are affectively experienced and given meaning. The following ethnographic accounts demonstrate how affectivity operates between the binary oppositions of cognitive and affective, intentional and unintentional. They illuminate how an intensity of verbal articulation about biological relatedness to the enemy give meaning to what 'I always felt . . . always knew', and recast the view on childhood experiences, providing a new understanding of parents as not simply despotic, cruel and emotionally withdrawn.

Marieke: I was never held or kissed by my mother, though I clearly remember she often kissed my younger brother. It was not only that I was much older than the brother who followed me (five years), but I always felt everyone in my family treated me like I was different . . . like a stranger. When my dad was angry with my mom, he would call her an 'Indisch whore'. I was not sure what that meant but I knew it was a 'bad word'. When he was angry with me, he would often say that I was 'just like my mom'. I suppose I made that connection on some level. I was bad and unworthy. I was so, so, *sooooo* shy; so ashamed of myself for a reason I could not explain. [Marieke, Indisch-Japanese woman, emphasis in speech]

Maarten: My father would often get angry at me, sometimes even if I had just broken a glass, and shout, 'you slit-eyed bastard, you ruined my life'. I could not understand how I could have ruined his life by breaking a glass or doing something insignificant like that. I knew; I felt it in my body that something was wrong with me; that I was irreparably different. I was much darker than my other siblings, and you know, being dark in an Indisch family is not a good thing. I was a quiet child, mostly playing on my own or reading, trying to stay away from my family members. I knew I could have been made responsible for anything that went wrong. I was always somehow inadequate. I was a lonely child and I only felt safe when I was alone . . . hahaha [laughs nervously]. People need family to feel safe, but I needed to be away from my family to feel safe. I could not understand it back then, but you see, *I was the living image of the enemy*! [Maarten, Indisch-Japanese man, emphasis in speech]

Ron: I'm still ashamed to say this but my father was a very cruel man. I was a rebellious teenager, I can't deny that, and I deserved to be sanctioned, but he would beat me so severely and then he would bury me in the ground up to my waist in our back garden, and I'd stay there like that the whole night. It was many years later that I learned that this was how some prisoners were treated in the Japanese prison camps. My father was not very kind to his other children either, but he was more supportive and never so cruel to them. My mom and I were the main targets of his outrage. [Ron, Indisch-Japanese man]

Like most Indisch-Japanese children, Marieke, Maarten and Ron grew up not knowing that their biological father was a Japanese man. What prevails in Indisch-Japanese narratives of childhood is a deeply felt sense of shame, loneliness, guilt, inadequacy, and ultimate difference – a feeling of being a stranger within. Common Indisch vengeance and hatred towards the enemy was transferred onto the mothers and their children as a 'dark stain'; a stigma impressed on them, producing a strong sense of otherness, marginalisation and exclusion. Discussing the ghostly presence of the affective atmosphere that generated a sense of unsafety and insecurity experienced by Marieke, Maarten and Ron – an atmosphere consisting of physical abuse, stigmatisation and rejection for 'faults' and 'wrongdoings' that were beyond comprehension – it is useful to turn to scholarship about the ghostliness of war and the intergenerational transmission of trauma.

Sociologist Avery Gordon cogently argues that 'haunting' is neither pre-modern superstition nor individual psychosis, but an important sociological phenomenon (2008, p. xvi). For Gordon, haunting is an animated state through which unresolved and repressed social violence makes itself known (2008, p. xvi). In hauntings as a social phenomenon, a ghost is not only a missing or a dead person, but a figure deeply implicated in social life and crucial for the production of subjectivities and histories (2008, p. x). In their theory of transgenerational haunting, psychoanalysts Nicolas Abraham and Maria Torok have argued that ignorance of family secrets, falsification, and disregard for the past are fertile ground for the production of hauntings across generations (1994, p. 169). They conceptualise the unconscious as a 'crypt' – a space from where ancestral secrets are passed down to the descendants. Jacques Derrida has argued that 'the inhabitant of the crypt is always a living-dead, a dead entity we are perfectly willing to keep alive, but as dead, one we are willing to keep, as long as we keep it, within us, intact in any way save as living' (1986, p. 78). Feminist cultural critics concerned with 'second generation' Holocaust memory work argue that feelings of loss are often transmitted intergenerationally, and not necessarily through speech (Hirsch, 1997; Hirsch and Smith, 2002; Kuhn, 1995). While this scholarship provides useful insights into intergenerational transmission, it does not sufficiently address the potential for self-transformation of, nor creative, critical reflection on intergenerational transmission, discussed shortly.

For Marieke, the missing embodied sensation of being held or kissed by her mother – an affection that was available to her younger siblings – generated a sense of estrangement and lack of worthiness of affection. The spatiality of her birth was an important element in the affective assemblage as well. Unlike her brother, who was born in the Netherlands, she was born in the colonial Dutch East Indies – a geographical location that, in her family's narratives, featured as a place of war, forced expulsion, but also the idealised life of pre-war times (see Dragojlovic, 2014). The affective power of the verbal abuse directed towards her mother ('Indisch whore') that demarcated her mother as an inappropriate and inadequate woman implicitly resonated with Marieke when she was labelled by the angry voice of her father as being 'just like your mother'. Believing that she was born in the early years of the Japanese occupation (1943), several months after her mother's husband was taken to the Japanese internment camp, Marieke developed the sense that she had done something wrong:

> After I was born everything went wrong in my family, in the colony. It is sad really, but every time I heard people lament the loss of the Dutch East Indies, I'd instantaneously feel this urgent panic in my body, like 'oh what have I done?' It sounds strange, but I lived with that feeling for many decades.

Marieke's experience of intergenerational suffering is constituted by distress caused by a lack of embodied parental affection, verbal abuse, a sense of shame for not being able to comprehend reasons for being treated differently and for not being able to forge a satisfying connection with her family members, and the spatial elements of a distant geographical location that ceased to exist as a unit (the colonial empire) as well as the discourses of loss associated with it. Here, we can see that the intensities of shame cannot and should not be defined as either 'cultural' or 'psychological' (see also Probyn, 2005, p. 7) but rather situated in ongoing gender inequalities and forces of structural racism. Thus, the intergenerational assemblages of suffering should not be seen as only revolving around an individual 'I' and that 'I''s family relations, but rather as inextricably linked to Indisch and especially Indisch-Japanese collective intergenerational suffering.

In her book *Haunting the Korean Diaspora* (2008), Grace Cho offers a nuanced analysis of the intergenerational transmission of memory. Her focus is on *yanggongju* – Korean women who acted as sex workers for US servicemen in Korea and who subsequently became war brides, pioneering Korean migration to the USA. Cho's careful analysis reveals how systematic erasure – an enforced forgetting of *yanggongju* – permeates the consciousness of the Korean diaspora. She argues that the *yanggongju* becomes a bearer of secrets about Korean War traumas; a ghostly figure that is at the same time present and absent, and 'moves in and out of visibility' (2008, p. 14). Cho's emphasis on the 'diasporic unconscious' is important for this discussion as it is not limited to the singular subject but rather situated through intersections of histories. As in Cho's work, in the Indisch-Japanese context, we see the forcible erasure of biological Japanese fathers that persisted until at least the 1990s, but that never left the 'diasporic unconscious'.

The materiality of broken glasses or dropped cutlery and the sound associated with those events resonate as embodied memories in Maarten's everyday life: 'Every time I hear things break or crackle like the glasses or other things [accidently broke in his childhood], I get agitated and upset.' The racialised verbal abuse Maarten received ('slit-eyed bastard') reiterates historical forms of racialization in which the Dutch colonial superiority was cast through discourses about Japanese and other Asian peoples as inferior to Europeans. Historical traces of structural racism reverberate as affective traces in Indisch-Japanese intergenerational suffering. For Maarten, as for many of the other Indisch-Japanese interlocutors (see also Ezawa, 2015), family and the family home did not feature as places of safety and protection – indeed, quite the opposite. Ron's embodied experience of being half-buried in the ground as a punishment and left as such overnight in the back garden of the family home constituted a major childhood trauma for him. At the time, he did not have knowledge about his biological relatedness to a Japanese man:

> I only knew that the man who I thought was my father hated me, and of course I hated him in return. It was many years later that I realised that he was not just punishing me, but also getting back at those Japanese men who had tortured him in the camp.

Here, affective states are imbricated into racialised associations of cruelty and ethnicity (the guards in the Japanese camps), fathers' embodied experiences of torture in the camps, and an association that Indisch-Japanese children carry the 'cruel essence' and mentality of their biological fathers. Based on the ethnographic material presented thus far, we can see how assemblages of human bodies, matters and things, cultural, gendered, social and racial discourses emanate as affective forces of intergenerational suffering wherein the subjective articulation is a crucially important aspect of self-contestation of the self.

The affective power of public articulation and restoration of the practice of secrecy

Well into the 1980s, narratives about Indisch-Japanese offspring remained outside of the Dutch public discussions. In 1983, two women fathered by a Japanese man during the Second World War placed an advertisement in one of the major Dutch newspapers, asking other people with similar genealogical links to join them in establishing a 'Japanese roots' group. Evelin Buchheim (2007, pp. 263–264) writes that only six people replied to this initial advertisement, but the following year, one of the descendants published her life story under a pseudonym in a book detailing the experiences of Indisch women in the Japanese internment camps. Shortly after the publication of that book, several members of the Japanese roots group shared their life stories on a national radio station. Following this public talk, the front door of one of the members was besmirched with the inscription '*hara-kiri*' (a Japanese term for ritual suicide) (ibid.). During the 1990s, the life narratives of Indisch-Japanese descendants began to feature regularly in the Dutch media, and in 2003, a prominent space was dedicated to Indisch-Japanese presentations at the *Pasar Malam*. Also during the 1990s, two organisations for Indisch-Japanese descendants were formed. The Association of Japanese-Indisch Descendants (*Vereniging JIN, Japans Indische Nakomelingen*) (JIN) was formed in 1991, and the Sakura Foundation (*Stichting Sakura*) was formed in 1995. Initially, both organisations had the aim of being a support network for people of similar descent.

The establishment of these organisations resonates with the emergence of therapeutic discourse in the 1980s, which postulates that the particularities of the past need both articulation and public revelation for the healing process to occur. Nicolas Rose (1990) refers to this as a rise of 'psy discourse', arguing that therapeutic culture has spread far beyond the medical therapeutic realms to become present in the sphere of everyday life. Similarly, Eva Illouz (2008) argues that 'therapeutic persuasion' has been institutionalised in many aspects of social life – from mass media and educational systems, to corporations. An important component of 'therapeutic persuasion' has been an emphasis on the confessional; the public revelation of dark secrets that has been most prominently present in television talk shows. To some extent, initiatives by both JIN and the Sakura Foundation are resonant with such 'therapeutic persuasion'. Yet, they are also self-reflexive engagements with the affective atmospheres in which Indisch-Japanese descendants grew up. These engagements are characterised by a deeply felt sense of knowing (a 'gut feeling') that something about them was different but was not, and could not be, openly articulated. Here, the practice of secrecy by those around the descendants operate as a moral, affective economy of caring. Actions by JIN and the Sakura Foundation and their members strive to speak to the 'diasporic unconscious' (see Cho, 2008), aiming to unearth and destabilise the relations and practices of secrecy that surrounded their birth and their lives prior to the disclosure about their Japanese descent. Yet, as will be discussed later in the chapter, such engagements are also complicit with prior moral values of caring.

Over the course of our conversations, Marianne (Akiko), who has been an active member of JIN for many years, stressed that the main aim of the organisation, and her personal one as well, was to:

> find all Indisch-Japanese children. There are many, many of us, but some people still do not know; others are still ashamed or they do not want to pass this information to their children or grandchildren. But that is wrong thinking.

Your children or grandchildren need to know their true roots; they need to know they are also Japanese, not just Dutch and Indisch. Such a secret cannot be kept forever, and it is never easy to deal with the fact that your father or grandfather was in the Japanese army, even when these were loving relationships. Like my mom – she had pictures of my dad, but had to burn them all after the war. My dad also gave me a Japanese name, Akiko. It is a beautiful name, isn't it? But you know, everybody hated the Japanese after the war, and I was not officially given that name. [Marianne (Akiko), Indisch-Japanese woman]

The necessity for open knowledge about Japanese descent that Marianne passionately argues for is part of a broader discourse advanced by many Indisch-Japanese descendants. Such discourses and practices of care (for those who do not know yet, or for future generations) in many ways represent a shift in moral values ascribed to productive caring relations. Yet, we suggest that, while discourses and practices of care that are focused on verbal articulation about biological relatedness and their affective economies (as advocated by JIN and Sakura Foundation and their members and affiliates) represent a shift in the notion of care, they do not discontinue the practice of secrecy. Similarly, while verbal articulation certainly brings about major self-contestations for Indisch-Japanese descendants, this does not mean that this form of care produces productive or harmonious relations. Open articulation and revelation prompt the shifting of elements within the affective assemblage, often with the effect of re-constitution of normative understandings of love and family, and thus social and biological reproduction. It should be noted, however, that such shifts often generate re-racialisation or anxiety for Indisch-Japanese family members. In other words, while elements of the assemblage shift and change with different affective intensity, the ethnographic material demonstrates that they remain intractably linked to valuing gender normativity and reinforcing the power of structural racism. This is best illustrated by the narrative of Marianne (Akiko)'s son, Jaap. When Dragojlovic first met Akiko in 2010, Jaap did not want to know anything about his mother's past and his Japanese grandfather. When Dragojlovic visited them in 2014, however, the son's interest and attitudes had changed significantly:

Jaap: It was a big thing really. Like, I never even identified as Indisch – my father is just an ordinary [white] Dutchman, and we thought my mom was only one quarter Indisch. She was always very close with one of her sisters who lives here in Rotterdam like us, but was not really close with the rest of the family, that lives in the south. They are sort of complicated . . . I do not know . . . We never socialised with them much. Then my grandfather fell ill and told my mom that he was not her real dad, but rather that some Japanese man was. That was very, very hard on my mom. She managed at first but then she collapsed. Soon she was diagnosed with depression! Why didn't they tell her earlier? It would have been easier on all of us. It's been two years now. She has made friends with some of the

JIN members, and that has helped. I tried to help her; I read a lot about the war years, about Japanese culture. I wanted to look at the good things about Japan. It was also important for me. It all came out of the blue – you are just told you are partly Japanese . . . it is very strange. My mom is better now, but we are still in sort of a shock, really. Look, it's fine with me. It's not like after the War. I think the Japanese are great; great technology, I love Manga comics. But look at me – so pale and blond – who'd ever believe me that my grandfather was Japanese? Haha. My girlfriend asked me the other day if I'd tell my children about my grandfather. Well, I don't know. I do not think it would matter to my children. Sometimes it is better to leave the past alone. [Jaap, Dutch, Indisch and Japanese man; the son of an Indisch-Japanese woman]

Paying attention to what affective assemblages do, we can see from Jaap's narrative that moral values of care are deeply informed by cultural and racial hierarchies, which echo the moral values that existed in the post-war years, as well as practices of secrecy. Here, however, the lack of disclosure about biological relatedness from the past is characterised as bad affect ('It would have been easier on all of us'), while a similar intention to downplay the importance of biological relatedness for future generations ('Sometimes it is better to leave the past alone') is reproduced as a caring relation (the virtue of forgetting). While both Jaap and Miranda's daughter (who is also 'white and blond') are clearly affected, they see themselves (in Jaap's case) and are seen by others (in Miranda's case) not only as having the potential to conceal information about their biological relatedness due to their light skin tone, but also consider this concealment as something that they should do ('leave the past alone').

Roots tourism and their affective potential

In this section, we explore how critical reflection on the practice of secrecy as a *moral economy of caring* and active engagement with the medical diagnostics of depression and burnout can generate self-transformation. Such transformation is enabled by affective assemblage of discourses, matters and things, medical diagnostics, and the ongoing effects of structural racism. In 2014, Dragojlovic visited Kim, who had told her via email communication that he had completely recovered from the severe burnout he had suffered some years earlier after finding out about the particularities of his adoption and biological relatedness. Entering his apartment on a quiet Sunday afternoon, Dragojlovic noticed that it had changed considerably since she had visited him for the first time several years earlier; Kim was very eager to show her the change. For him, the change to his apartment demonstrated his departure from his depressive states, wherein physical objects and matters stand as important elements in the affective assemblage of transformation. The living room was entirely redecorated in Japanese-style furniture he had obtained in the Netherlands. Similarly, his library was filled with books about Japan and his walls were decorated with calligraphic paintings brought from

Japan, as well as framed prints of haiku poetry. Next, Kim proudly showed his kitchen, where he had been spending a lot of time perfecting his Japanese cooking, using what he referred to as 'original' recipes and ingredients brought back from Japan. Kim was curious to know if Dragojlovic could detect how his body language had changed; he told her that after several visits to Japan and some prolonged stays in the country, his friends and relatives had noticed it. He had even more been often taken for a 'real Japanese' person while in Japan.

During his severe burnout, Kim's wife found out about JIN, and Kim immediately joined this organisation. Being in the position to share and compare experiences with other Indisch-Japanese descendants for the first time in his life brought Kim a sense of relief from, and resolution to the depressive state he had been experiencing. Soon after joining, Kim went on a 'roots tour' to Japan, which is one of the main activities of the JIN organisation (see also Buchheim, 2015). The following narrative is how Kim described his shifting emotions towards Japan and his affective experience of visiting the country, which had brought about major shifts in his life. He shared this account with Dragojlovic after performing a 'traditional Japanese tea ceremony' he had learned during one of his visits.

My whole life, I have been avoiding all things Japanese: Japanese culture, Japanese language, learning about Japanese war, *my FACE!* When I first moved to Amsterdam and noticed that Japanese tourists regularly tried to talk to me in Japanese, I started to avoid touristy places on purpose. I even avoided Japan in my studies. I specialised in regional relations in Southeast Asian countries, and Japan has a role there, but I did not want to know anything about the Japanese. I first started learning Chinese because *Japanese was too hot for me; I could not bear it!* But that whole thing broke down once I went to Japan for the first time.

Uuuuuuuuu . . . that was something . . . uuuuuu . . . really big. I had lived my whole life in a white environment but in Japan, people looked like me!!! Since I do not know anything about my Japanese father, I could not look for him, but just being in Japan changed everything for me. *It gave me life again!* Ever since my first visit in 2008, I have been visiting Japan on an annual basis. I have friends there and I feel good about it.

What I have discovered over the years is that there was another story in my family I did not know anything about. My biological mother had a sister who had a very good relationship with a Japanese man and they wanted to marry each other. They were planning to migrate to Brazil, but it did not happen. This aunt lives in California now. She migrated there with her son and married again. I learned about her existence only after I got so depressed; people in my family thought that getting in touch with her might help. I contacted her and she was very open to talk about it because she had a child of her own born to a Japanese father, like me. I told her about the JIN and she joined it, too.

JIN started looking for her son's biological father and found a family living in Kumamoto, but the man had already passed away. When I went to Japan, I visited Kumamoto, hoping to meet my cousin's half-siblings. I sent them a letter and met a half-brother and that was nice. While they knew about each other, my cousin in California was not interested in this at all. I visited him in California, but unlike here, over there it is so multiracial that he does not need to chase his Japanese half-siblings; he belongs to California. Hahah . . . There are many Asians living there. There are also second-generation Japanese people who, like me, do not speak Japanese. But, unlike me, my cousin has no need to learn about Japanese history or culture. He knew all his life that his father was Japanese and it was not a problem over there like it was in the Netherlands.

Kim's genealogy work is a practice of self-exploration and self-making (Basu, 2006; Dragojlovic, 2011, 2014; Kramer 2011; Nash, 2008; Saar, 2002); an integrative element of the intergenerational suffering assemblage through which he seeks self-transformation. As we can see in his narrative, the self is not prescribed or given, but rather in a continuous process of becoming. The self is fluid and provisional, pointing towards personal fragility emanating from the structural force of the intersectional inequalities caused by postcolonialism, racism, and sexism.

Conclusion

The ethnographic material discussed in this chapter has demonstrated a need to reconceptualise suffering as historically embedded and intergenerationally located. Here, secrecy about biological relatedness to the enemy soldier causes emotional distress across generations. We have also seen that the public revelation of secrecy does not necessarily elevate suffering beyond that secrecy, and instead can lead to the restoration of the practice of secrecy, leaving open questions about the future and whether the ongoing practice of secrecy will be complicit in ongoing suffering in the future. We have argued that hauntings are a useful conceptual way of capturing the presence of intergenerational presence of unhappy affect, often lived as suffering, but a question remains as to whether, and if so how, such affective forces will continue in the future. In the case of Indisch-Japanese descendants, biological relatedness is seen as unimportant (seen in the adoption practices and concealment of biological relatedness in the aftermath of the Second World War). At the same time, though, the practice of secrecy surrounding it emanates as an affective, moral economy of caring, reinforced by heterosexual normativity and the effects of structural racism that reverberate across generations. The ethnographic material presented in this chapter challenges the idea that the effects of historical violence are located in a singular body, with a clear demarcation between articulation and silence, and between healthy and ill bodies. Rather, it stresses the importance of paying attention to how intergenerational distress is shaped, constituted, contested, transformed and sustained as an affective assemblage of suffering. The ethnographic material we analyse here is best approached as an affective assemblage that changes in form and intensity over time. Thus, these assemblages are open-ended and malleable, yet also specific to historical contingencies.

In this chapter, we have worked towards a theoretical conceptualisation of intergenerational suffering as affective assemblages, to think *with* experiences of historical violence and the practice of secrecy beyond the binary oppositions of conscious and unconscious, intentional and non-intentional, mind and body, health and illness, culture and psychology. Thus, the affective assemblages are constitutive of disparate elements: human bodies, things and matters, embodied memories of physical pain that exceed the boundaries of a singular body, shame, exclusion, marginalisation, love, distress, compassion. As such, focusing the analysis on the affective assemblages allows us to move away from situating suffering and distress in relation to historical violence and forced displacement within the binary oppositions of social and cultural, embodied and somatic, ill and healthy bodies. This focus also enables the exploration of processes of continual becoming and the potential for ongoing self-transformation.

Thus, the historical violence and its ghostly reverberation over time cannot be limited to a simple understanding of a body's capacity 'to affect and be affected' (e.g. Massumi, 2002). Rather, it needs to be situated within particular historical contingencies, wherein the affectivity of historical violence reverberates through assemblages of immaterial affects (Blackman, 2012, pp. 173–174) discourses, practices and performance-shaping subjective formations. The ethnographic material discussed here alerts us to the need to re-conceptualise our understanding of intergenerational suffering caused by multifaceted forms of violence and marginalisation, whether historical (imprisonment in Japanese camps, effects of restrictive gender norms, forced migration) or contemporary (racialisation, perpetuation of ideals of normative family and love). Thus, intergenerational suffering must be understood beyond personal psychopathologies, and we must turn our attention to the fragility of the embodied individual and collective selves. So doing, this chapter makes a contribution to the emerging body of scholarship that argues for the exploration of the productive and transformative possibilities of negative feelings, 'failure' and suffering (Blackman, 2015; Cvetkovich, 2012; Davies, 2012; Halberstam, 2011), while stressing the affective intensities of intergenerational suffering embedded in the moral economy of caring.

Notes

1 Several edited volumes have been dedicated to collections of case studies about war children born out of sexual violence (e.g. Carpenter, 2007, 2010; Grieg, 2001).
2 For a genealogy of trauma, see Leys (2013); for a critical discussion, see Fassin and Rechtman (2009); Hacking (1995); Young (1996).
3 Instead of these paradigms, Kidron (2009, p. 18) examines how survivors' homes embed the presence of the Holocaust through silent and embodied practices, which she argues are 'nontraumatic lived memory'. Basing her claim on her interlocutors' arguments that they were not suffering from the effects of transmitted trauma, Kidron normalises her interlocutors' nightmares and episodes of weeping as 'lived memory . . . within the everyday private social milieu' (ibid., p. 3).
4 For detailed discussions of the affective capacity of the environment, see Dragojlovic (2015); Navaro-Yashin (2012); Thrift (2008). For a discussion of the affective capacity of matter, see Bennet (2010).

5 For the Australian context, see, for example, Coté and Westerbeek-Veld (2005) and Duyker (1987); for the Netherlands, see Pattynama (2000).
6 In anthropology, secrecy has been studied particularly in relation to secret society. Mahmud (2014) provides a detailed overview of this area of study.

References

Abraham, N. & Torok, M. (1994). *The Shell and the Kernel: Renewals of Psychoanalysis*. Chicago: University of Chicago Press.
Ahmed, S. (2004). Affective economies. *Social Text*, 79(22), pp. 117–139.
Ahmed, S. (2010). *The Promise of Happiness*. Durham, NC: Duke University Press.
Argenti, N. & Schramm, K., eds. (2010). *Remembering Violence: Anthropological Perspectives on Intergenerational Transmission*. New York, Oxford: Berghahn Books.
Basu, P. (2006). *Highland Homecomings: Genealogy and Heritage Tourism in the Scottish Diaspora*. New York: Routledge.
Blackman, L. (2012). *Immaterial Bodies: Affect, Embodiment, Mediation*. Thousand Oaks, CA: Sage.
Blackman, L. (2015). Affective politics, debility and hearing voices: towards a feminist politics of ordinary suffering. *Feminist Review*, 111(4), pp. 25–41.
Bosma, U. & Raben, R. (2008). *Being 'Dutch' in the Indies. A History of Creolisation and Empire, 1500–1920*. Singapore and Ohio: Singapore University Press and Ohio University Press.
Buchheim, E. (2007). 'Hide and seek': Children of Japanese-Indisch parents. In Blackburn, K. & Hack, K., eds, *Forgotten Captives in Japanese-occupied Asia*. Abingdon and New York: Routledge, pp. 260–277.
Buchheim, E. (2015). Enabling remembrance: Japanese-Indisch descendants visit Japan. *History & Memory*, 27(2), pp. 104–125.
Butler, J. (2005). *Giving an Account of Oneself*. New York: Fordham University Press.
Carpenter, R. C., ed. (2007). *Born of War: Protecting Children of Sexual Violence Survivors in Conflict Zones*. Bloomfield: Kumarian.
Carpenter, R. C., ed. (2010). *Forgetting Children Born of War: Setting the Human Rights Agenda in Bosnia and Beyond*. New York: Columbia University Press.
Cho, G. M. (2008). *Haunting the Korean Diaspora: Shame, Secrecy, and the Forgotten War*. Minneapolis, MN: University of Minnesota Press.
Connerton, P. (1989). *How Societies Remember*. Cambridge: Cambridge University Press.
Coté, J. and Westerbeek-Veld, L. (2005). Recalling the Indies: Colonial Culture and Postcolonial Identities. Amsterdam: Aksant.
Crapanzano, V. (2011). *The Harkis: The Wound That Never Heals*. Chicago: University of Chicago Press.
Csordas, J. T. (2008). Intersubjectivity and intercorporeality. *Subjectivity*, 22, pp. 110–121.
Cvetkovich, A. (2012). *Depression: A Public Feeling*. Durham, NC: Duke University Press.
Danieli, Y., ed. (2010). *International Handbook of Multigenerational Legacies of Trauma*. New York: Plenum Press.
Davies, J. (2012). *The Importance of Suffering: The Value and Meaning of Emotional Discontent*. London, New York: Routledge.
Davoine, F. & Gaudilliere, J. M. (2004). *History Beyond Trauma*. New York: Other Press.

de Jong, L. (2002). *The Collapse of a Colonial Society: The Dutch in Indonesia during the Second World War*. Leiden: KITLV.

Deleuze, G. & Guattari, F. (1987). *A Thousand Plateaus: Capitalism and Schizophrenia*. Minneapolis: University of Minnesota Press.

Derrida, J. (1986). Foreword: Fors: The Anglish words of Nicolas Abraham and Maria Torok. In Abraham, N. & Torok, M., *The Wolf Man's Magic Word: A Cryptonymy*. Minnesota: University of Minnesota Press, pp. xi–il.

Derrida, J. (1994). *Specters of Marx: The State of The Debt, the Work of Mourning, and the New International*. New York: Routledge.

Derrida, J. (2001). *A Taste for the Secret*. London: Polity.

Dragojlovic, A. (2011). 'Did you Know my Father?': the zone of unspeakability as postcolonial legacy. *Australian Feminist Studies*, 69(26), pp. 317–332.

Dragojlovic, A. (2014). The search for sensuous geographies of absence: Indisch mediation of loss. *Bijdragen tot de Taal-, Land- en Volkenkunde* (*Journal of the Humanities and Social Sciences of Southeast Asia*), 170(4), pp. 473–503.

Dragojlovic, A. (2015a). Hunted by miscegenation: gender, the white Australian policy and the construction of Indisch family narratives. *Journal of Intercultural Studies*, 36(1), pp. 54–70.

Dragojlovic, A. (2015b). Affective geographies: Intergenerational hauntings, bodily affectivity and multiracial subjectivities. *Subjectivity*, 8, pp. 315–334.

Dragojlovic, A. (2016). Playing family: Unruly relationality, and transnational motherhood. *Gender, Place and Culture: Journal of Feminist Geography*, 23(2), pp. 243–256.

Duyker, E. (1987). *The Dutch in Australia*. Melbourne: ae Press.

Ericsson, K. & Simonsen, E., eds. (2005). *Children of World War II: The Hidden Enemy Legacy*. Oxford: Berg.

Eyerman, R. (2002). *Cultural Trauma: Slavery and the Formation of African American Identity*. Cambridge: Cambridge University Press.

Ezawa, A. (2015). 'The guilty feeling that you exist': War, racism and Indisch-Japanese identity formation. In Kowner, R. & Demel, W., eds., *Race and Racism in Modern East Asia: Interactions, Nationalism, Gender and Lineage*. Leiden and Boston: Brill, pp. 481–502.

Fassin, D. & Rechtman, R. (2009). *The Empire of Trauma: An Inquiry into the Condition of Victimhood*. Princeton, NC: Princeton University Press.

Feuchtwang, S. (2011). *After the Event: The Transmission of Grievous Loss in Germany, China and Taiwan*. New York: Berghahn Books.

Gordon, A. (2008). *Ghostly Matters: Haunting and the Sociological Imagination*. Minneapolis, MN: University of Minnesota Press.

Grieg, K. (2001). *The War Children of the World*. Bergen: War and Children Identity Project.

Hacking, I. (1995). *Rewriting the Soul: Multiple Personality and the Sciences of Memory*. Princeton, NJ: Princeton University Press.

Halberstam, J. J. (2011). *The Queer Art of Failure*. Durham, NC: Duke University Press

Hirsch, M. (1997). *Family Frames: Photography, Narrative and Postmemory*. Cambridge and London: Harvard University Press.

Hirsch, Marianne (2008). The generation of postmemory. *Poetics Today*, 29(1): 103–128.

Hirsch, M. and Smith, V. (2002). Feminism and cultural memory: An introduction. *Signs*, 28(1), pp. 1–19.

Hoffman, E. (2010). The long afterlife of loss. In Radstone, S. & Schwarz, B., eds, *Memory: Histories, Theories, Debates*. New York: Fordham University Press, pp. 406–415.

Illouz, E. (2008). *Saving the Modern Soul: Therapy, Emotions, and the Culture of Self-Help*. Berkeley, CA: University of California Press.

Kidron, C. (2009). Toward an ethnography of silence: The lived presence of the past in the everyday life of holocaust trauma survivors and their descendants in Israel. *Current Anthropology*, 50, pp. 5–27.

Kidron, C. (2012). Breaching the wall of traumatic silence: Holocaust survivor and descendant person – object relations and the material transmission of the genocidal past. *Journal of Material Culture*, 17(1), pp. 3–12.

Kidron, C. (2010). Silent legacies of trauma: A comparative study of Cambodian Canadian and Israeli holocaust trauma descendant memory work. In Argenti, N. & Schramm, K., eds., *Remembering Violence: Anthropological Perspectives on Intergenerational Transmission*. New York and Oxford, Berghahn Books, pp. 193–229.

Kirmayer, L. J., Gone, J. P. & Moses, J. (2014). Rethinking historical trauma. *Transcultural Psychiatry*, 51(3), pp. 299–319.

Kramer, A.-M. (2011). Kinship, affinity and connectedness: Exploring the role of genealogy in personal lives. *Sociology*, 45(3), pp. 379–395.

Kuhn, A. (1995). *Family Secrets: Acts of Memory and Imagination*. London: Verso.

Leys, R. (2011). The turn to affect: A critique. *Critical Inquiry*, 37(3), pp. 434–472.

Leys, R. (2013). *Trauma: A Genealogy*. Chicago: University of Chicago Press.

Locher-Scholten, E. (1995). Veerwerking en koloniaal trauma. Balans van begrippen. *Bzzletin*, 24(228), pp. 3–9.

Love, H. (2007). *Feeling Backward: Loss and the Politics of Queer History*. Cambridge, MA: Harvard University Press.

Mahmud, L. (2014). *The Brotherhood of Freemason Sisters: Gender, Secrecy, and Fraternity in Italian Masonic Lodges*. Durham, NC: Duke University Press.

Massumi, B. (2002). *Parables for the Virtual: Movement, Affect, Sensation*. Durham, NC: Duke University Press.

Nash, C. (2008). *Of Irish Descent: Origin Stories, Genealogy, and the Politics of Belonging*. Syracuse: Syracuse University Press.

Navaro-Yashin, Y. (2012). *The Make-Believe Space: Affective Geography in a Postwar Polity*. Durham, NC: Duke University Press.

Pattynama, P. (2000). Assimilation and masquerade. Self-construction of Indo-Dutch women. *European Journal of Women's Studies*, 7, pp. 281–299.

Probyn, E. (2005). *Blush: Faces of Shame*. Minneapolis, MN: University of Minnesota Press.

Rose, N. (1990). *Governing the Soul: The Shaping of the Private Self*. London and New York: Routledge.

Saar, M. (2002) Genealogy and subjectivity. *European Journal of Philosophy*, 10(2), pp. 231–245.

Simmel, G. (1906). The sociology of secrecy and of secret societies. *American Journal of Sociology*, 11(4), pp. 441–498.

Stoler, A. L. (2002). *Carnal Knowledge and Imperial Power: Race and the Intimate in Colonial Rule*. Berkeley, CA: University of California Press.

Taussig, M. (1999). *Defacement: Public Secrecy and the Labor of the Negative*. Stanford, CA: Stanford University Press.

Taylor, J. (1983). *The Social World of Batavia: European and Eurasian in Dutch Asia*. Madison, WI: University of Wisconsin Press.

Thelen, T. (2015). Care as social organization: Creating, maintaining and dissolving significant relations. *Anthropological Theory*, 5(4), pp. 497–515.

Thrift, N. (2008). *Non-Representational Theory: Space, Politics, Affect*. New York: Routledge.

To, N. (2015). Diasporic montage and critical autoethnography: Mediated visions of inter-generational memory and the affective transmission of trauma. In Knudsen, B. T. and Stage, C., eds, *Affective Methodologies*. New York: Palgrave Macmillan, pp. 69–97.

Walkerdine, V. (2010). Communal beingness and affect: An exploration of trauma in an ex-industrial community. *Body & Society*, 16(1), pp. 91–116.

Yehuda, R. (2006). *Psychobiology of Posttraumatic Stress Disorder. A Decade of Progress.* Boston, MA: Blackwell.

Young, A. (1996). *The harmony of illusions: inventing post-traumatic stress disorder.* Princeton, NJ: Princeton University Press.

4 Racialisation and othering as everyday harm

Embodiment, adoption, affect

Following on from Chapter 3, this chapter further analyses suffering as an affective assemblage produced by racialisation, othering and the contested moral economy of caring at the level of family and society. Scholars have argued that under neoliberalism, suffering and 'feeling bad' have become 'ordinary' (Blackman, 2001, 2015; Cvetkovich, 2012) rather than being exceptional experiences, manifested through a sense of fear and anxiety about potential personal inadequacies, and a perception of failure to achieve the manifold expectations that are required for people to live 'happy' and 'successful' lives. Queer and feminist scholars discuss such workings of neoliberalism as 'happiness duty', manifested in affective and moral performances of happiness (Ahmed, 2010); as the 'tyranny of success' (Halberstam, 2011); and depressive states as its cultural and political phenomena (Cvetkovich, 2012). This series of happiness normativities in the contemporary milieu are manifested in the lives of many, but emerge as pernicious in the context of particular forms of othering and racialisation of transnational adoptees. The expectation that creating a family through transnational adoption will fulfil the image of a happy and successful family has, under neoliberalism, created a demand for knowledge about the health conditions of potential adoptees (Herman, 2008). This 'adoption medicine' creates categories of adoptees' bodies – that is, healthy, ill, abled – and reveals a prevailing desire for healthy, able-bodied children (van Wichelen, 2014).

Here, as in the rest of the book, our conceptualisation of suffering as affective assemblages is focused on the exploration of how the expectation of harmonious, happy families and grateful, content and successful adoptees intersects with the long history of racialisation and ethnicisation of the non-white 'other' in the Netherlands. We have done this by focusing on the experiences of non-white adoptees who had been raised in white families. Our analysis is based on ethnographic data collected by Dragojlovic in the Netherlands in 2013–2014 with adult adoptees who had been brought together by adoptee support group, *For Adoptees*.[1] The group was established by a number of adoptees who had a mission of representing, protecting and defending the needs of adoptees. Ever since its establishment, *For Adoptees* has been run as a safe space where attendees can openly and self-reflectively engage with experiences of negative feelings (unhappiness, shame, depression, failure, anxiety, low self-esteem, suicidal tendencies, rage, self-harm) and the diagnoses of psychological disorders some of them have been given. Importantly, the group is only open to adoptees, and not to their other adoptive family members. The group name – *For Adoptees* – relates to different aspects of adoptees' lives, corresponding with, first, the *mobility* that occurs through transnational adoption; second, the presumed, imagined, and contested notion of *abandonment* by an adoptee's biological parent(s), which is commonly a source of adoptees' ponderings and often part of the reasoning in the pathologisation of their feelings; third, *adaptation and assimilation*, which is seen as necessary for their incorporation into their white families; and lastly, *affection*, wherein the psychopathologisation of adoptees' bodies postulates that adoptees are susceptible to developing attachment disorder.

Starting from the premise that adult adoptees' interests, needs and feelings need to be supported and protected, *For Adoptees* has, since its conception, engaged in different forms of affective politics that challenge the psychopathologisation of adoptees' negative feelings, and addressed the everyday harm that racialisation and othering has on non-white bodies. We foreground the political in the everyday life experiences of adoptees by paying attention to the immediate, and personal, rather than perceiving the political as that which occurs solely in the public life of the community (e.g. Arendt, 1958). Moreover, we also explore how the adoptees' community is un-made, and contested through affective politics. This provides another way of thinking about the undulations of suffering.

In this chapter, we ethnographically explore the modalities of the affective politics in which *For Adoptees* engages, in order to inquire into what such engagements allow adoptees to do and become. Our analysis builds on queer, feminist and critical race scholarship that productively engages with negative feelings not in terms of pathology (Ahmed, 2010; Blackman, 2015; Cvetkovich, 2012; Halberstam, 2011; Love, 2007), 'nor distinctly toxic' (Sedgwick, 1993, p. 63) but rather as capable of having creative and productive ends. In this way, we seek to explore how affective politics and subject formations resist normative demands and strive to cultivate social change. We argue that thinking about suffering under the neoliberal framework – that is, as being 'ordinary' rather than exceptional – might divert our attention from how the structural force of the intersectional inequalities caused by postcolonialism, racism and sexism can generate everyday harm and suffering to non-white bodies in the Netherlands – a society that imagines itself as white (Wekker, 2016). We explore how *For Adoptees'* affective politics mobilise the adoptees' negative feelings as a form of resistance against the normative demands that affect adoptees' subjecthoods, wherein adoptees are expected to feel like grateful, successful and content citizens. We explore how these normative demands are produced by the dominant power structures of whiteness, normative family values and the sexualisation of non-white bodies. Furthermore, this chapter explores how therapy cultures that are commonly understood to work towards the normativisation of emotions and the production of happy subjects (e.g. Berlant, 2011; Illouz, 2008; Rose, 1990) can have a subversive potential in their active mobilisation of negative affect and the value they ascribe to negative feelings. This provides another layer of nuance to our argument around suffering as affective assemblages of bodies, technologies, discourses, practices and performances.

The transformation of family life

Over the last three decades, transnational adoption has become a global phenomenon, and families formed through transnational adoption have emerged as one of many manifestations of the transformation of the traditional, nuclear family, consisting of parents and their biological children.[2] Beginning in the 1960s on the backdrop of declining birth rates in the United States and countries of Western Europe, transnational adoption became a common way of forming a family for involuntarily infertile couples. Since these beginnings, transnational adoption has seen children being adopted mainly from Asia (Korea, China, Vietnam, Thailand, Cambodia, the Philippines, Taiwan, Indonesia, India, Sri Lanka, Bangladesh), South America (Columbia, Chile, Brazil, Peru, Honduras, Haiti, Mexico, El Salvador, Guatemala), Africa (Ethiopia, South Africa) and from the former Russian republics and other eastern European countries (e.g. Howell, 2009; Hübinette, 2004; Yngvesson, 2010).

This new way of forming families has been defined as 'kinning' by Norwegian anthropologist Signe Howell. Howell uses this term to describe 'the process by which a foetus or new-born child (or a previously unconnected person) is brought into a significant and permanent relationship with a group of people that is expressed in a kin idiom' (Howell, 2003, p. 465). Through this process of kinning, adoptees' bodies, which are treated as blank slates, become incorporated into their adopted families. In the first several decades of transnational adoption, adoptees were legally disconnected from their pre-adoptive pasts and incorporated into their adoptive families and nations 'as if' they had been born there (De Graeve, 2015; Yngvesson, 2012). This approach was based on the notion that adoptees (non-white in white families) would be smoothly incorporated into their adoptive families as well as their new countries' languages and cultures. Strongly postulated on the idea that their adopted middle-class white families would 'erase' their 'otherness', such an approach completely undermined the significance of the racialisation of the international adoptees (e.g. De Graeve, 2015; Hübinette, 2004; Hübinette and Tigervall, 2009; van Wichelen, 2015). Indeed, adoptees' sense of non-belonging is frequently framed in psychological terms, attributed to such conditions as attachment disorder and the early trauma of having been abandoned or otherwise separated from their biological kin (De Graeve, 2015). Similarly, much of the extensive psychological literature on adoption focuses on the formation of adoptees' identities through the lenses of behavioural and mental health problems (e.g. Brodzinsky et al., 1990).

Our analysis builds on, and diverges from this scholarship in several ways. First, our analytical lens is focused on how members of *For Adoptees* who grew up as non-white adoptees in white families self-reflectively engage with their own psychological diagnostics, psychological scholarship that analyses adoptees' bodies through the framework of behavioural and mental health problems, in conjunction with the narratives of their everyday experiences of racialisation and othering. Thus, our ethnographic material urges us not to make a clear demarcation between psychological diagnostics and the societal circumstances that cause adoptees' experiences of everyday suffering.

Second, we explore how ongoing attempts to simultaneously erase and reinforce the otherness of non-white adoptees in white families (within a society that imagines itself as white are normalised through discourses and practices of care and caring. Thus, we introduce the concept of *everyday harm*, which emanates from non-intentional affects that emanate from and are reinforced by normative understandings of family, loyalty and relatedness, and the effects of structural racism on non-white bodies. The ethnographic material demonstrates that *everyday harm* is closely related to the *moral economy of caring*, and that it cautions us against presuming that care necessarily produces harmonious relations. As in Chapter 3, we explore how the complex set of moral obligations to care for children and, in this case, for cultures from which children have been adopted, often produce unhappy affect.

Third, we ethnographically explore how *For Adoptees* attendees engage with drawings, photographs, and academic and popular texts about adoption in their self-reflective engagements with their own negative feelings. To achieve what this book aims to do – that is, examine suffering as being constituted by affective assemblages – we further engage in the problematisation of the human body as a bounded, singular entity (Blackman, 2012; Mol, 2002). We also consider how human bodies, matters and things, discourses, performances and practices collide. This is part of our aim to explore how experiences of everyday harm are shaped, contested and sustained.

As in the rest of the book, we argue for an understanding of human suffering as an affective assemblage by focusing our analysis on *what assemblages do* (Deleuze & Guattari, 1987, p. 257) and on the capacity of assemblages to transform. Thus, we ethnographically explore how racialisation and othering emanate as affective assemblages of suffering that operate through and across the binary oppositions of cognitive and affective, intentional and non-intentional. Further, we offer a critique of the banishment of the subject from affect studies, and argue that attention must be paid to how affectivity is racialised, gendered, qualified and given meaning by the subject; and how affectivity is central for understanding ongoing processes of becoming (see also Blackman, 2012; Navaro-Yashin, 2012). This is important, as it alerts us to how engaging with negative feelings through affective politics can open up creative and productive possibilities. In this way, subjects can be inspired and encouraged to resist the normative demands imposed on them (adoptees) and their subjecthood, and to strive for the kind of social transformation wherein non-white bodies are not racialised or othered.[3] As in Chapter 3, by considering how adoptees self-reflexively engage with negative feelings, we call for a reconsideration of the entrenched idea that emotional suffering primarily emanates from a singular human body, and argue that negative feelings should not necessarily be primarily understood within the parameters of an individual's psychopathology.

The ethnographic setting

This chapter is based on ethnographic research conducted with adult adoptees brought together by the support group *For Adoptees*. Since the 1960s, approximately 50,000 children have been adopted into the Netherlands, including around 5000 from China, 4400 from Columbia, 4100 from South Korea, as well as around 25,000 from within the Netherlands itself (Hoksbergen, 2011). The Netherlands has one of the highest per capita rates of international adoption in the world, with only Norway, Sweden, Denmark, Switzerland, France and Canada having higher rates (Selman, 2002). It is estimated that more than 30,000 transnational adoptees – mainly from Asia and Latin America – live in the Netherlands (Hoksbergen, 2011). *For Adoptees* is open to all adult adoptees, regardless of their country of origin. As such, both transnational and domestic adoptees have been in attendance at the group's meetings, but it is predominantly the transnational adoptees who regularly attend. This appears to be mostly due to the fact that the topics discussed at *For Adoptees'* gatherings tend to relate to racialisation and othering of non-white bodies. Over the past ten years, around 200 adoptees have attended *For Adoptees'* meetings, which usually last around three hours, and cost 30€ each.

Dragojlvoic met *For Adoptees'* leader, Daniel,[4] in 2010 while conducting research on Indisch memory and genealogy work (see Dragojlovic, 2011, 2014, 2015a, b). Together with a group of Indisch memory workers, Daniel has trained as an integrative psychotherapist, Family Constellation therapist[5] and personal/ life coach. Daniel, like Dragojlovic's other Indisch interlocutors (see Chapter 3), was concerned with exploring the contested sense of non-belonging that had emanated through their lives. In the case of adoptees, they described this as non-white bodies being moved (without their consent) to a predominantly white society. After experiencing 'burnout' in his late 30s, accompanied by dissatisfaction with his romantic relationships (characterised by repeated breakups rather than the longevity he desired) and a psychological diagnosis of attachment disorder, Daniel began to explore what he referred to as 'adoptees' condition'. When Dragojlovic first met him, Daniel had been working as a life coach and therapist for three years, having abandoned his work as a human resources manager in a multinational company. Hearing about Dragojlovic's interest in memory and genealogy work in relation to forced mobility and historical violence, Daniel, who conceived of transnational adoption as a form of forced mobility, was eager for Dragojlovic to conduct research on adoptees, and offered to share his time and to introduce her to his broad network of adoptee clients, friends and acquaintances. Accepting his invitation, Dragojlovic conducted semi-structured interviews and had numerous open-ended conversations with 37 adoptees. During this period, Dragojlovic attended several *For Adoptees* group meetings and Family Constellation healing workshops, and took part in many informal social events attended by adoptees and their family members and friends. Most of Dragojlovic's interlocutors were adoptees from Korea, though several were from Bangladesh, Haiti, Ethiopia, and three had been adopted from and within the Netherlands.

Some of the *For Adoptees* attendees Dragojlovic came into contact with had experienced ongoing feelings of unhappiness, shame, depression, failure, anxiety, low self-esteem, suicidal tendencies, rage and self-harm, and had, at various stages in their lives, been diagnosed with an anxiety disorder. Many of these attendees were dissatisfied with the effects of the psychotropic medications that had been prescribed to them, and with the psychological counselling they received. Others described their interest in attending *For Adoptees'* meetings as stemming from wanting to understand their contested feelings of non-belonging, and were engaging with those feelings through what we refer to as *identity work* – an active exploration of the self that is primarily focused on understanding how to deal with everyday experiences of racialisation and othering. For many of the attendees, attendance at these meetings constituted a search for understanding and an attempt to contextualise the negative feelings they had been experiencing; a method of finding ways to verbally articulate feelings that are known and familiar (shame, guilt, low self-esteem, anger, etc.) but lack discursive articulation.

The driving force behind the establishment of *For Adoptees* was the dissatisfaction that Daniel and several other adoptees (some of whom had trained as psychologists, psychotherapists and social workers) had felt about the psychological diagnoses they had been given, which they considered had been focused only on the 'abandonment' they had experienced from their biological mothers and the early childhood trauma that this abandonment had presumably produced. According to *For Adoptees'* organisers, much of the psychological therapy to which they had been exposed did not discuss their adoptive parents or engage with the dynamics that had existed in the families they had grown up in. Neither this nor the general racialisation that exists in Dutch society, it seemed, were considered to be important components or factors in their emotional distress. Instead, the diagnoses were predominantly focused on the adoptees as being 'failed' individuals, with this failure seemingly unrelated to their adoption and subsequent incorporation into a predominantly white society.

Adoptees who had disconnected from their adopted families in adolescence or adulthood had a strong sense that they were, as a consequence, continuously shamed by people in broader society (such as acquaintances, work colleagues and neighbours), and were characterised as ungrateful and disrespectful towards their adoptive parents, who had 'saved them'. At the same time, the parenting of the adoptive parents was never questioned. There was rising concern among the organisers of *For Adoptees* about the high rates of attempted and successful suicide that existed among their adoptee friends and family members, which, they argued, others simply saw as further evidence of the 'failures' of the adoptees to fit into Dutch society and culture. Initially, the *For Adoptees* support group was established to provide a safe place where adoptees could share their experiences openly, without feeling marginalised or dismissed if their attitudes and experiences did not fit into the idealised notions that surrounded adoption in the

Netherlands, consisting of caring parents and grateful adoptees. In addition to this, the organisers provided the group with counselling, guidance and supervision. Over the years, the attendees changed, and under the initiative of Daniel and some new therapists who joined the group, the group's also changed, to include discussions of academic writings written by, and art produced by adoptees about their experiences of growing up as non-white bodies in white families. In effect, this new focus was on actively engaging with residual feelings of being different, beyond the psychological paradigm of personality disorders. Many attendees of *For Adoptees* meetings were trained social workers, psychologists, life coaches and psychotherapists. Some had been trained in these professions prior to joining the *For Adoptees*, but many had embarked on these new professions after attending *For Adoptees*' sessions.

In what follows, we first offer a broad literature review on transnational adoption by paying specific attention to the scholarly work that was used as reading material by the attendees of *For Adoptees*. This is followed by a detailed ethnographic exploration of how affective politics are practised and how and what kind of atmosphere is produced by the narratives shared and matters discussed at *For Adoptees*' gatherings. Finally, we suggest that the meetings enabled critical reflection about the everyday harm the adoptees suffered, which was caused by the racialisation and othering, but also open critical spaces for problematising relations of care. In this section, we analyse the use of subjective transformation as a resisting force against the normative demands of adoptees' subjecthood.

Transnational adoption

With the dramatic increase in transnational adoption over the last 30 years, academic writings on the topic have proliferated, predominantly within the fields of anthropology (e.g. Carsten, 2007; Howell, 2009; Kim, 2010; Volkman, 2005; Yngvesson 2010), psychology (e.g. Hjern et al., 2002; Lindblad et al., 2003, von Borczyskowski et al., 2006) and interdisciplinary fields spanning gender studies, critical race studies and human geography (Castañeda, 2011; De Graeve, 2015; Leinaweaver & van Wichelen, 2015; Van Wichelen, 2015; Walton, 2015). Emphasising the centrality of spatiality to belonging and the importance of racialisation in transnational adoption, an emerging body of interdisciplinary, comparative scholarship conceptualises transnational adoption through the lens of geographies of migration and childhood (Leinaweaver & van Wichelen, 2015). As a detailed review of scholarly literature on adoption is beyond the scope of this chapter, we instead offer detailed information about the scholarly work that was closely read, and much debated, by the *For Adoptees* support group's members.

Most of Dragojlovic's interlocutors grew up at a time when the prevailing adoption practices in the Netherlands approached adoptees as blank slates who would be easily incorporated into both their adopted families and into Dutch national culture. As such, more recent adoption discourses that stress the paradigm of 'the rooted child' and the importance of adoptees having a connection to their countries of birth (De Graeve, 2015; Jacobson, 2008; Marre, 2007; Volkman, 2003; Yngvesson, 2010) remained out of the discussions at *For Adoptees*.

Familiar with scholarly literature about adoption, Daniel, along with several other psychologists, psychotherapists and social workers involved in the group, stressed the importance of understanding the difference in academic writings about adoption between, on the one hand, those produced by academics who are adoptive parents, and, on the other, by academics who are adoptees themselves. This viewpoint has also been emphasised in scholarship produced by adoptees (e.g. Walton, 2015). Daniel made this distinction for Dragojlovic, to aid her in her work as a researcher, but also emphasised this to his clients and to *For Adoptees* attendees. The idea that priority should be given to scholarship produced by adoptees rather than adoptive parents was accepted unanimously, but discussion about the arguments produced in such scholarly work were points of heated debate, as we discuss in the following section.

One of the books that featured prominently for many of the Korean adoptees in *For Adoptees* was *International Korean Adoption: A fifty-year history of policy and practice* (Bergquist et al., 2007). This text was written by adoptees, and was often referred to as an important part of Korean adoptees' collective history. Other important reading material in the group was Indigo Willing's (2006, 2009) discussion about racialisation in adoption practices in the Australian context. However, by far the most read, debated and contested work was that of Tobias Hübinette (2004, 2007) and his collaborator Carina Tigervall (2009). Across his publications, Hübinette offers a trenched critique of transnational adoption practices in general (2007), and about adoption in Sweden in particular (Hübinette & Tigervall, 2009). Positioning his work within the field of postcolonial theory and critical race studies, Hübinette is particularly interested in the effects of everyday racism and the Orientalist imaginary that positions Asian children as quiet, kind, hard-working, docile and submissive (ibid., p. 2007). He argues that, unlike in the US, the ideology of colour-blindness in Scandinavia postulates that there is no racism outside of right-wing extremism. Even though more recent studies focusing on Sweden have demonstrated widespread discrimination and racism towards migrants and other minorities, the prevalent national imagery in Sweden is that of a non-racist country. Despite very different national histories and the Netherlands' long history of colonialism, the Dutch national imagery is (like in Sweden) one of colour-blindness and negation of the existence of racism and racialisation (see Dragojlovic 2016a; Essed & Hoving, 2014; Wekker, 2016). Hübinette's critiques have resonated closely with *For Adoptees* members, and have provided them with a sense of commonality with adoptees who grew up in Sweden.

Aside from the recognition of and importance ascribed to the everyday racialisation of non-white adoptees, what drew most of Dragojlovic's interlocutors towards Hübinette's and Tigervall's (2009) work is the attention this work gives to the results of quantitative psychological studies conducted in Sweden about adoptees. Given that *For Adoptees* was formed to some extent as a critical response to the anxiety and personality disorders many of the initial group members were diagnosed with, it seems somewhat unexpected that Dragojlovic's interlocutors would be interested in the results of quantitative psychological research. The results (which were published in English) were read by many *For Adoptees* members with great interest. The quantitative research concluded that adoptees have the highest attempt and accomplishment rate of suicide in Swedish society. This is four to five times higher than the rates seen in any other demographic subgroup. The researchers also argued that adoptees in Sweden are more susceptible than immigrant groups to alcohol and drug abuse, criminality, psychiatric illnesses, being overweight and experiencing significant problems in attaining their adoptive parents' socioeconomic status (Hjern et al., 2002; Johansson-Kark et. al, 2002; Lindblad et al., 2003; von Borczyskowski et al., 2006). While urging scholars and practitioners to take the results of this research into serious consideration, Hübinette and Tigervall (2009) argue that the results should not be seen only as reflecting the problems of particular individuals. Rather, these results should be considered against the backdrop of the ongoing racialisation of non-white adoptees that occurs not only within Swedish society at large, but also within the adoptees' families.

Many *For Adoptees* members have, at one point or another in their lives, experienced intense feelings of homelessness, loneliness, fear of abandonment, guilt, melancholia, heightened sensitivity to disapproval and criticism, suicidal and depressive tendencies, unexplainable panic attacks and intense interpersonal relationships (alternating between extremes of idealisation and devaluation). These members have been diagnosed with depression, chronic depression, borderline personality disorder, attachment disorder, attention deficit hyperactivity disorder (ADHD), or bipolar disorder. This, combined with their adoptee friends and acquaintances having had similar experiences (including, in some cases, having friends who had committed suicide), sheds some light on the reasons why the members and attendees of *For Adoptees* took the Swedish psychological research into adoptees so seriously. *For Adoptees* members were well aware of the emotional distress they and other adoptees had experienced, but struggled to locate such distress within the psychological paradigm of personality disorders. Agreeing with Hübinette (2004, 2007) and Hübinette and Tigervall (2009), Dragojlovic's interlocutors argued that psychological research needed to include other aspects of adoptees' experiences of everyday life, as discussed in the following section.[6]

Radical affective politics

In this section, we focus on two meetings of the *For Adoptees* support group. In the first meeting discussed below, the aim was to provoke a discussion about everyday racism by engaging in a heated debate about whether transnational adoption can be compared with slavery, and whether non-white adoptees bodies are 'disembedded' and 'out of place'. In the second meeting, the focus was on discussing the experience of growing up in white families as non-white adoptees, by exploring visual images produced by adoptee artists. The images included drawings in the satirical children's book entitled *The Bastard Nation Bed Time Stories*, and a series of photographs featuring young adoptees holding banners presenting sayings and presumptions pertaining to everyday experiences of racialisation and othering of non-white adoptees growing up in white families. These materials were produced by adoptee activists.

'Disembedded' and 'out of place' bodies?

The first *For Adoptees* meeting discussed in this chapter gathered 20 people and was described as a session to discuss the body and embodiment. At the opening of the meeting, several participants shared stories of their most recent everyday encounters, in which they had had to prove that they were 'regular Dutch people' to those who (based on the appearance of their non-white bodies) linked them to other places and cultures. Tom, a man in his mid-30s who had been attending the *For Adoptees* sessions for some time and who had been having regular counselling sessions with Daniel, stated firmly that 'there has not been a single day in my life in which I was not taken for an Antillean man'. By this, Tom meant that he is perpetually being taken for a black migrant man from the Netherlands Antilles, a location that is often associated, in Dutch public discourses and state policies, with criminality (van Amersfoort & van Niekerk, 2006). Here, racialisation operates as a normalised and unproblematic association between place and race (see also Dragojlovic, 2015; Razack, 2002).

Daniel stressed that adoptees' bodies have been removed from their countries without their consent, and possibly without willingness on the parts of their biological parents to give them away. Being adopted from Korea at the age of four, Daniel remembered his biological mother's sadness and how he cried for her when he was brought to his new family in the Netherlands. Daniel was adopted in the early 1970s as the seventh adopted child (of an ultimate total of nine) into a family of devoted Protestants living in a small country town in the Netherlands. Daniel often referred to his adopted parents as having adopted 'rainbow children' (from Indonesia, India, Brazil, Ethiopia and Korea) as an expression of their religious humanitarianism. In such a family, religious devotion and expressing gratitude for having been 'saved' were expected of all the adopted children.

Prior to the meeting that day, Daniel had distributed an article written by Tobias Hübinette (2007) to the attendees of *For Adoptees*, entitled 'Disembedded and free-floating bodies out-of-place and out-of-control: Examining the borderline existence of adopted Koreans'. Daniel invited the attendees to comment on it at the meeting. Carmen, a woman in her late 30s who had been adopted from Korea when she was three months of age, and who grew up in a family with two younger siblings (one also adopted from Korea, and the second, a biological child of her adopted parents), commented that she had enjoyed reading the article and agreed with the problematic nature of racialisation, but also noted that she also found some of the comparisons drawn between transnational adoption and slavery to be too harsh and unconvincing. Repeating her agreement with the article, that adoptees are often unproblematically racialised within their own families, she reminded us of her name, which had been given to her in homage to the main protagonist from the opera *Carmen* by the French composer Georges Bizet, which her adoptive parents had liked. Carmen remembered her parents saying while she was growing up that her hair was just like Carmen's – black and long. When Carmen saw images of the Carmen from the opera, she became aware that she did not look like Carmen at all:

> She had big brown eyes; she was white and beautiful, and I have slit eyes and I thought, 'my parents must be so disappointed with me, I'm nothing like the real Carmen . . .' I was ashamed of myself. It was very hard for me. Still, I can't really think about my parents as malicious racists. They named me after their favourite opera character. They were loving and caring.

Carmen described her adoptive parents as leftist liberals who were concerned about the injustices in the world, and who understood the practice of adoption as a way of saving 'abandoned' and 'unwanted' children. 'There is nothing wrong with people wanting to help others, care for others . . . Only, the way your parents care for you can hurt you.' Natalie, who had also been adopted from Korea, commented that she agreed with Hübinette that many Korean adoptees were perceived as kind, hard-working, often passive and obedient. Yet, Natalie did not see that perception as being a problem. In fact, she was convinced that such personality traits were inherently Korean; something that would have stayed with her regardless of where or in which family she had grown up. To that, Tom replied:

> You might be right, but I do not feel like a rough and tough black man from the Caribbean. People see me like that – even my in-laws can't think of me differently. It is fine if you feel like a hard-working Asian, but that is a stereotype. It is all the damned colonialism, my dear friend.

The agitation in Tom's voice was followed by a brief silence. The silence was interrupted by Natalie, who replied: 'I suppose there is a difference between Asian and Black people.' Tom sighed loudly and left the room.

Being critical of transnational adoption in general, and keen to discuss the most potentially controversial aspects of the practice, Daniel began to comment that, thus far, international adoption agencies have transported at least half a million children from the global South to the global North in a period of 50 years (he was quoting from Hübinette, 2007, p. 135). As such, he continued, transnational adoption has many similarities with Atlantic slavery and with contemporary trafficking in women for sexual exploitation and international marriage market. Daniel then read the following passage from Hübinette's text:

> Both the slaves and the adoptees are separated from their parents, siblings, and relatives as an early age; stripped of their original cultures and language; reborn at harbours and airports; Christianized; re-baptized and given the

name of their master, and in the end retained only a racialized, non-white body that has been branded or given a case number.

(Hübinette, 2007, p. 135)

'This is not just Tobias,' he continued. As far back as 1986, scholar Igor Koptyoff realised that there were similarities in commodification between adoptees and slaves (Hübinette, 2007, p. 135). At this point, Ineke (who had been adopted from Korea in 1983 as a 2-month-old) interrupted Daniel in a passionate, loud voice:

> This is nonsense! We are *not* slaves! I have a good life here, my parents care for me . . . You do not want to see how bad Koreans are. If they had cared for us, they would not have given us away! You are so bitter about the Dutch and your adopted parents, but that does not give you the right to call me *slave*! I am Dutch! Nothing else! [emphasis in speech]

Countering Hübinette and Daniel's interpretation of it, Ineke argued that, based on her own readings and her degree in cultural studies from the one of the most prestigious Dutch universities, Hübinette's argument was incorrect and that he should have read more about hybridity and postcolonial theory. Amelia (a woman in her mid-30s who had been adopted from India as a 4-month-old) commented in a calm voice, 'if everything is so great for you here Ineke, what brought you to this discussion? You told us last time you were diagnosed with a chronic depression?' Ineke replied in as agitated a manner as before:

> You people think all the problems you have in life are related to adoption. 'Poor adoptees' [she said in a sarcastic voice]. Stop thinking about yourselves as victims! Go and live! So what if people think I am from somewhere else? Well, I was born in Korea, they did not care about me over there and good people who cared took me to live with them here. I am not ashamed of having been adopted. Get over your shame!

After making her point, Ineke took her coat and bag and left the room, loudly slamming the door on her way out. A long silence followed, and Daniel suggested we take a break and have some tea and biscuits. The session did not resume on a group level, but people continued to chat in small groups. Moving from group to group, the participants were heard almost unanimously agreeing that Ineke's reaction stemmed from her having been given up for adoption and her struggle to engage with effects of racialisation. The other attendees said Ineke knew this 'deep down', that 'she sees it in the mirror she is not white'; 'she feels in her body she is different. It pains her, we have all been there'; 'she'll come again. What she feels but cannot say will not stop bothering her.'

Here, it is useful to focus our discussion on the affective atmosphere and affective dynamic of this *For Adoptees* meeting. Almost without exception, the attendees of this meeting knew prior to coming that these meetings are always 'intense', 'emotional', 'hard' and potentially 'upsetting' due the topics covered. Yet, it was precisely the potential affective intensity and discursive engagements of the meetings that was being sought here. *For Adoptees* engages in what we call 'radical affect politics', which is expressed through an intentional engagement with what has been silenced (effects of everyday racism and othering), pathologised (unhappiness, depression, rage, pain, suicidal tendencies, self-harm) and marginalised (any resistance to the normative demands of adoptees' subjecthood, e.g. adoptees refusing to perform the role of a loyal and dutiful adopted child). By engaging with these negative feelings, the adoptees were seeking to articulate and contextualise the world both within and outside of their adopted families, as well as within broader circles of friends and acquaintances and the psychological diagnostics process.

Most of the attendees at the *For Adoptees* meetings seek to de-pathologise these negative feelings and, through such engagements, seek new forms of attachment (among the group members, both during and outside of the meetings) as well as support and encouragement to cultivate subject positions that resist the normative demands of adoptees' subjecthoods. Thus, attendees arrive at the meetings with the intention of experiencing an intense affective atmosphere. This is not to say that all meetings have the same intensity. On the contrary, some were described as 'un-uneventful', 'fine', or/and 'the usual' (narrating experiences of everyday racialisation). In her seminal work on the transmission of affect, Teresa Brennan (2004) describes 'how one feels . . . the "atmosphere"' and argues that such analysis needs:

> to take accounts of physiology as well as the social, psychological factors that generate the atmosphere in the first place. The transmission of affect, whether it is grief, anxiety, or anger, is social or psychological in origin . . . the transmission is also responsible for bodily changes; some are brief changes, as in whiff of the room's atmosphere, some longer lasting. . . . The "atmosphere" or the environment literally gets into the individual.
>
> (Brennan 2004, p. 1)

Brennan's argument stems from her critique of psychoanalysis, which conceives of affect as primarily emanating from the interiority of the human subject. She convincingly challenges the subject–object divide by proposing a focus on what she refers to as 'affective transfer' among human subjects and between humans and their environment (see also Navaro-Yashin, 2012). Several other scholars approach affective atmospheres as experiences that occur across human and non-human bodies, beyond the subject–object distinction, and before and alongside subjective formations (Anderson, 2009; Anderson & Wylie, 2009, Dragojlovic 2015b; Seigworth, 2003). Yet, neither bodies nor atmosphere exist as neutral or stable entities. Rather, they are generated through specific affective relations between human bodies, matters, things, discourses and practices.

Thus, the affective intensities of the *For Adoptees* meeting discussed here are both intentional and non-intentional, cognitive and non-cognitive, as well as largely dependent on the material discussed and the people in attendance, as well as these people's own attitudes, feelings, medical conditions and life-stages (e.g. if they were first-comers to the meetings, if they were going through a particularly difficult period in their lives, if they had just made their first visit to their country of birth or had just met their biological parents and/or siblings). The ethnographic material from this meeting urges us not to approach affect as only an outside stimulus that is non-intentional, pre-subjective and non-cognitive (Clough, 2007; Massumi, 2002; Thrift, 2008), but rather as intensities that circulate between human bodies, matters and things that are subjectively experienced (see also Blackman, 2012; Dragojlovic, 2014; Knudsen & Stage, 2015; Leys, 2011a, b; Navaro-Yashin, 2012) and must be socially, politically and historically situated.

The affective intensities and dynamics brought about by the readings of Hübinette's text and the specifically situated lives of those who attended the meeting – being affectively reminded of naming as a practice or racialisation (Carmen), contesting the relationship between racial hierarchies and individual traits (Tom and Natalie) – poignantly highlighted how normative power structures of whiteness and racialised hierarchies re-incited feelings of distress, anger, rage and contested loyalty. We can see how the affective economy of racialisation, normalised through 400 years of Dutch imperial rule, makes whiteness appear 'normal . . . [and] devoid of meaning' (Wekker, 2016, p. 2), while non-white bodies are understood to embody difference. In a context where the dominant national narrative postulates that racism does not exist in the Netherlands and where such a misconception is often articulated through zealous, forceful and oftentimes aggressive denials (Dragojlovic, 2016; Essed & Hoving, 2014; Wekker, 2016), articulating the effects of racialisation on non-white bodies is often a difficult and challenging task.

For many adoptees who attended the *For Adoptees* meeting, coming to terms with the fact that they had been othered and racialised was a difficult process that, for many, took years and often meant being perceived as a 'trouble maker', a 'failure' or an 'ungrateful child' by their adopted families and oftentimes their acquaintances and friends. In her recent study on the paradoxes of colonialism and racism in the Netherlands, Gloria Wekker (2016) persuasively demonstrates that the collective Dutch self-imagery of what is 'non-Dutch' includes such characteristics as 'language, an exotic appearance . . . outlandish dress and convictions . . . the memory of oppression' (ibid., p. 7). As part of this self-imagery, these characteristics are expected to be shed away as fast as possible by new arrivals who have non-white Dutch ancestry – 'all signs of being from elsewhere should be erased' (ibid., p. 7). The dominant representation of Dutchness as whiteness, monoethnicism, and monoculturalism dates back to the standardisation of Dutch language and culture that took place in the end of the nineteenth century (Lucassen & Penninx, 1993; Wekker, 2016). Thus, claiming rightful belonging to the Dutch nation for those of darker skin tones is an ongoing, everyday task, challenged by everyday assumptions that associate non-white bodies with foreignness and otherness.

The day following the heated discussion at the *For Adoptees* meeting, Dragojlovic was having lunch with Daniel and Carmen. Carmen was telling us her plans for her next visit to Korea, where she was going with her two children and her husband. In the middle of our conversation, Daniel's phone rang and, explaining that he had to take the call, he answered it and left the table. Carmen went on to tell Dragojlovic about her degree in applied psychology, which she was due to complete in June that year. Re-joining them almost half an hour later, Daniel seemed exhausted. He sat down with a sigh of relief and informed Carmen and Dragojlovic that he had been speaking to Ineke, who was angry about the previous day's meeting. Ineke criticised his practice as a life coach and therapist, telling him that what he was saying about adoptees was nonsense; that he was trying to brainwash people about being subjected to racism, that racism does not exist in the Netherlands, and that he was trying to convince the adoptees that they were victims. Carmen commented, with a sense of empathy and compassion:

> It is hard for her. I remember, when I was younger, dreaming night after night that I was white, like the real Carmen, and in the morning I would face my Asian features in the mirror . . . It's painful for her, she does not want to accept what she already knows – that she is not white!

Daniel reiterated his statements that 'suffering is a part of life . . . a necessary way of learning, especially for non-white people in a white society. Antidepressants will not solve her problems.' Just like the other attendees of the *For Adoptees* meeting, Daniel and Carmen interpreted Ineke's reactions as a struggle to conceptualise her feelings as unhappiness caused by the normalisation of the racialisation of non-white bodies in the Netherlands.

In their conversations with Dragojlovic, Daniel and the group of psychologists, psychotherapists and social workers that work with him continually stressed the importance of engaging with feeling bad and suffering as an integral part of what it means to be human, rather than a psychiatric problem that requires medicalisation and antidepressant therapy. Instead, they have attempted to approach suffering as relational and as an emotion that needs to be perceived in the broader cultural and social context in which peoples' lives are situated. Thus, they do not see suffering as an emotion to be avoided or chemically altered, but rather to be self-reflectively engaged with.[7]

The *Bastard Nation Bed Time Stories*

The other *For Adoptees* meeting we discuss here examined satirical visual images about adoptees in order to encourage the adoptees to self-reflectively engage with the most painful forms of racialisation and othering they grew up with. The initiator of this activity was Carmen, who said that she clearly remembered that she never enjoyed her birthday parties as a child, but once she had her own daughter, started going to great lengths to organise the 'perfect celebration'. While her husband and the rest of the family were supportive of this idea, Carmen said:

> I was so obsessed with my daughter's birthday party that I could not sleep for days prior to the event. At some point, I told my friend that I needed to

relax about it a bit. She asked me about my own birthday parties, and I told her I did not like them, convincing her that adoptees in general do not like their birthday parties as it reminds us that we were abandoned. But my friend did not stop there. She kept asking, 'what were your parties like? Who was there? What did you do?' And that was a hard thing to remember! I could not clearly remember the people's faces, what we did, the birthday cake and such things. What I remembered were very loud, overwhelming voices saying, 'you must feel very lucky to live here', 'children are dying out of hunger in country where you were born', 'you are so lucky to have found such nice parents, so many children in Korea live in orphanages', 'you are born under a lucky star to live here', 'you should be very grateful to your parents who saved you from the orphanage, you should celebrate [your adoption] as your second birthday.' The voices went on and on in my head, they were so loud and horrible. Before I knew what was happening, I felt my friend's gentle hug and realised I was sobbing . . . See, that was so hard for me, that I had forgotten it; could not remember it. I had thought that disliking my birthdays had to do with abandonment, but there was something else there as well.

Carmen stumbled upon the blog, *The Daily Bastardette*,[8] which frequently features drawings for the covers of books of imaginary bedtime stories for adoptees under the name *Bastard Nation Bed Time Stories*. Reading over this blog, she recognised many of the statements that had had a profound effect on her growing up, but which she had never consciously reflected upon. This prompted Carmen to share the blog with the other attendees at the next *For Adoptees* meeting, and to make the blog a point of discussion. In response to this, the other attendees brought with them writings from the other blogs, mainly featuring statements of sayings that 'should never be told to an adoptee', as produced by adoptee activists. Carmen suggested that people split into pairs, take the images and statements, and try to rank them from one to ten, with 'one' representing the statement that affected them the most. The *Little Book of Adoption 'Truths'* featured the image of a little girl reading a book. Part of this image is covered by the following statements: 'you should be grateful'; 'you must be loyal'; 'if it weren't for us you would be alone'; 'it is your fault you do not fit in'; 'you were unwanted'; 'your mother loved you so much she abandoned you'; 'you are unlovable'; 'your origins are irrelevant'. The juxtaposition of this image with these statements invokes the kind of atmosphere in which these adoptees would have grown up.

Sayings that 'should never be told to an adoptee' were represented as photographs of young adoptees holding banners with the following statements: 'your mom is a real saint for wanting you'; 'she isn't your real sister, you know that'; 'you are lucky your parents came to save you, otherwise you would be dead on the streets'; 'it is so nice of your mom to save you'; 'your parents could have lived in a better suburb and travelled the world but they adopted the two of you'; 'why didn't her real family want her'; 'you are lucky you've got the pretty one' [to the parents]; 'she speaks really good Dutch'. Similar to the statements written in the *Bastard Nation Bed Time Stories*, these accounts depict the atmosphere of othering and racialisation of non-white adoptees that exists in their everyday lives. The images of young adoptees holding testimonials about their experiences work as a powerful affective force in reminding attendees of how they themselves were as children.

Soon after the material was exchanged, the room was filled with the sounds of deep sighs and soft and loud sobs. Mariane, who was born to an Ethiopian mother and a Dutch father and was adopted when she was 12 months old, had never seen any of the images or materials shared by the group and found herself profoundly affected by what she was seeing:

> This is me, this is me! All of it . . . all of it! I can't make a list of priorities, they are all important for me. The gratefulness, I always felt I needed to do more, to show them [her parents] that I am as good as their biological daughter. But birthdays, I hated them so much! I was so ashamed that my biological mother did not want me, it made me feel so different and somehow bad.

The attendees shared their experiences and comforted each other with words and long hugs. During the tea break, with which the session ended for that day, Rene (a woman in her late 30s who had been adopted from Korea as a 3-month-old) said:

> These meetings saved my life. They are hard, difficult, they dig deep into your soul, your body, into things you do not dare to think about yourself. But once you face them, you feel better. With the others here, I have a very strong bond. We understand each other. It is not that I do not have a good relationship with my adopted parents, but they are white. They were not adopted. They cannot understand what it means to be adopted . . . The way we [*For Adoptees* attendees] care for each other is priceless.

Like many other attendees, Rene valued the affective intensity of the meetings, and stressed their importance for her own self-transformation. The reactions of the other attendees and the meaning they assigned to the affectivity of the meetings show the attendees' willingness to engage with affective politics of the *For Adoptees* method, which encourages subjective transformation that challenges and rejects the normative expectations of adoptees' subjecthoods. At this meeting, the radical affective politics of *For Adoptees* was constituted by different elements: discourses about adoption, the effects of everyday racialisation, human and non-human bodies and technologies (the participants' bodies, as well as the printed works, the technology of academic writing, and the satirical drawings and slogans made by activist adoptees), as much as the performances enacted by the very existence of the *For Adoptees* meetings. Here, reading, looking at and commenting on satirical images serve as self-reflective ways of dismantling the affective economy of caring, which reinforces normative understandings of family, loyalty and relatedness.

We suggest that the affectivity of the visuality and materiality of the texts, their articulation, and the specific ideas they generate about adoptees' bodies and embodiment are all important elements of the affective assemblages, and illuminating of *what assemblages do* (Deleuze & Guattari, 1987, p. 257). They also show how assemblages of suffering, which emanate from the affective economy of racialistion and othering, can shift and transform. Blackman (2012, p. 134) and Blackman and Venn (2010) argue that approaching affect as the body's capacity to affect and be affected might be too broad, but note that this could be interpreted as a quality or vital element expressed though affect. Thus, the body is understood through connectivity and relationality, rather than through a separation of mind from the body, and human from non-human. Yet, based on the ethnographic material discussed in this chapter, which showcases the affective atmosphere at the *For Adoptees* meetings, we argue that the body's capacity 'to affect and be affected'[9] needs to be situated within specific historical contingencies, prevailing structural racism and normative understandings of family and loyalty.

The discussions that occurred during the *For Adoptees* meetings demonstrate how the *moral economy of caring* is multidimensional, destabilising the idea that care for others produces harmonious relations. Rather than being approached as uni-directional (Thelen, 2015), the relationship of care between care givers (parents) and care receivers (children) needs to be approached as multifaceted. As such, attention must be paid to the tensions and power relations that exist within relations of care, rather than assume that caring intentions and the relations they produce are a stabilising force. Work in the field of critical disability studies emphasises the importance of paying attention to power relations within the relations of care, and stresses that care can limit the personal autonomy of care receivers (Watson et al., 2004; Williams, 2001).

Conclusion

Scholars have argued that therapy cultures work to normalise and normativise emotions (e.g. Berlant, 2011; Illouz, 2008; Rose, 1990). Yet, the ethnographic material we have discussed here highlights the subversive potential of what can broadly be termed 'therapy culture' by actively engaging with, and valuing experiences of negative feelings. *For Adoptees*' practice of 'radical affect politics' reveals the creative possibilities of questioning the normative demands posed on adoptees' subjecthoods, and problematises the normalisation of care relations (in this case, adoption) as being harmonious and devoid of power relations. The ethnographic material has shown that non-white adoptees' bodies are perceived as embodying distant cultural geographies, and resonates with the following argument from Goldberg: 'Just as spatial distances like "West" and "East" are racialised in their conception and application, so racial categories have been variously spatialised more or less since their inscription' (1993, p. 185). Such racialised categories and their implied hierarchies echo in non-white adoptees' experiences of growing up in white families and living in a society that imagines itself as white, and manifest themselves as everyday experiences of harm and suffering that are often elusive and difficult to articulate. Thus, we argue that rather than approaching suffering under neoliberalism as 'ordinary', we must pay attention to how the structural force of the intersectional inequalities caused by postcolonialism, racism and sexism can generate everyday harm and suffering. We emphasise the need to attend to the specificities of suffering as reinforced by normative expectations of happy and harmonious families, demonstrating how these expectations generate particular forms of suffering in everyday experiences. We argue for neoliberalism to be seen as a messy, diffused part of the overall assemblage of suffering in the contemporary world.

Having as its main goal the 'empowerment' of adoptees, which will allow them to be 'who they really are' – individuals able to voice their negative feelings without being pathologised for it or made to feel like failed, ungrateful citizens – the leaders of the *For Adoptees* support group engage in the therapeutic method of radical affective politics which intentionally attempts to generate an affective atmosphere charged with feelings of pain, suffering, hurt and discomfort, aiming to provoke attendees into confronting and challenging the harmful forces of everyday racism and othering that surround them. In other words, *For Adoptees'* radical affective politics mobilise the re-production of negative feelings in its subjects, aiming to cultivate a resistance within them against the normative demands imposed upon their subjecthoods. These demands require them to be grateful, successful and content citizens and are produced by dominant power structures of whiteness, normative family values of the non-white bodies. The methods employed by *For Adoptees* and practised by their attendees urges us to see the human body not as a singular, bounded entity, but as always linked to other bodies, whether human or non-human, including technologies, matters and things (Blackman 2012; Mol, 2002). We are also led to see bodies as in a process of ongoing transformation. Thus, as in Chapter 3, we call for the reconsideration of the idea that emotional suffering primarily emanates from the individual human body, and argue that negative feelings should not primarily be understood within parameters of individual psychopathology.

How does this add to our overall understanding of suffering in its idiosyncrasies, but also as a broader social experience? One key aspect revealed here is the pernicious character of the placement and concealment of negative affect in neoliberalism – the banishment of that which is 'unhappy', 'pessimistic' or 'troubled' from the realm of the desirable, virtuous and valued. These normative structures are ubiquitous, but induce considerable suffering among those who are othered or marginalised through everyday racism. Therapy offers the possibility of release from negative affect, and of recognition of collective harm and suffering, challenging notions of separateness, togetherness and the 'wounded' person, and instead reconstituting the collectivity of harm, and the diffuse and personal character of suffering.

While such dynamics are specific to the group/s in which they exist, they are also reflective of the social fabric, and ripple effects, of neoliberalism. Therapy is made necessary by the normative virtue of happiness, the illusion of individual responsibility and the cultural desire and requirement for optimism (even within trauma). These factors force us to conceal the negative aspects of our (individual and collective) experiences and the affective dimensions that conflict with the requirements of forms of power and authority. This presents as an important case study in the broader rejection of pain as being located securely within the person, rather than being located (or rippling) across people; and of the illusion that the pursuit of normality, healthy citizenship, optimism and individual togetherness is a pernicious facet of our cultural milieu. This distracts the onlooker from the realisation that, in fact, a person's experience and their suffering emerges from the atmospheres of othering, sexism, racism and collective violence. Once again, through this exploration, we reiterate that suffering does not take place in a vacuum. Instead, humans are subjects of our times; active players and disciplined subjects of the expectations of our cultural milieus. Most importantly, our personal troubles are collective problems, and the denial of negative affectivity is part of this (new) disciplinarity. To disrupt this denial, as groups such as *For Adoptees* do, is to challenge the very nature of where suffering is located, how it lingers, and how it may be cast away.

Notes

1 The name of the group and its attendees, as well as the names of all sites and location, have been altered in order to protect the anonymity of my interlocutors.
2 Yet, despite changes that have been occurring, the heteronormative, middle class, white nuclear family is still understood as a model against which other families are measured up against (e.g. Dragojlovic, 2016a; Kawash, 2011; Seidman, 2004).
3 Lisa Blackman (2015) makes a compelling argument for feminist futures that are attentive to the negative states of being, and for intertwined relations between politics, emotions and affects.
4 Throughout the text, we have used pseudonyms in order to protect the privacy of our interlocutors.
5 Family Constellation Therapy is an alternative therapeutic method that was developed by German psychotherapist Bert Hellinger in the 1980s. This method will be discussed in greater detail in Chapter 5.
6 During Dragojlovic's ethnographic research at the *For Adoptees* meetings, psychological research on the behavioural and mental health of the adoptees in the Netherlands was not discussed. Some of the attendees referred to the work of Wendy Tieman (2006).
7 Such an approach in many ways echoes the work of the British anthropologist and psychotherapist James Davies, as is developed in his book *The Importance of Suffering* (2012).
8 See www.dailybastardette.com/bastard-nation-bedtime-stories-flippingthe-script-on-the-adoptee-narrative/.
9 On the body's capacity 'to affect and be affected', see also Massumi (2002).

References

Ahmed, S. (2010). *The Promise of Happiness*. Durham, NC: Duke University Press.
Anderson, B. (2009). Affective atmospheres. *Emotion, Space and Society*, 2(2), pp. 77–81.
Anderson, B. & Wylie, J. (2009). On geography and materiality. *Environment and Planning A*, 41(2), pp. 318–335.
Arendt, H. (1958). *The Human Condition*. Chicago: University of Chicago Press.
Bergquist, K. J. S. et al., eds. (2007). *International Korean Adoption: A Fifty-Year History of Policy and Practice*. New York: Haworth Press.

Berlant, L. G. (2011). *Cruel Optimism*. Durham, NC: Duke University Press.

Blackman, L. (2001). *Hearing Voices: Embodiment and Experience*. London and New York: Free Association Books.

Blackman, L. (2012). *Immaterial Bodies: Affect, Embodiment, Mediation*. Thousand Oaks, CA: Sage.

Blackman, L. (2015). Affective politics, debility and hearing voices: Towards a feminist politics of ordinary suffering. *Feminist Review*, 111(4), pp. 25–41.

Blackman, L. & Venn, C. (2010). Affect. *Body & Society*, 16(1), pp. 1–6.

Brennan, T. (2004). *The Transmission of Affect*. New York and London: Cornell University Press.

Brodzinsky, D. M. & Schechter, M. D., eds. (1990). *The Psychology of Adoption*. Oxford: Oxford University Press.

Carsten, J. (2000). *Cultures of Relatedness: New Approaches to the Study of Kinship*. Cambridge, Cambridge University Press.

Carsten, J. (2007). Constitutive knowledge: Tracing trajectories of information in new contexts of relatedness. *Anthropological Quarterly*, 80(2), pp. 403–426.

Castañeda, C. (2002) *Figurations: Child, Bodies, Worlds*. Durham, NC: Duke University Press.

Castañeda, C. (2011). Adopting technologies: Producing race in trans-racial adoption. *The Scholar and Feminist Online*, 9, pp. 1–5.

Clough, P. T. (2007). Introduction. In Clough, P. T., with Halley, J., eds, *The Affective Turn: Theorizing the Social*. Durham, NC, Duke University Press, pp. 1–34.

Cvetkovich, A. (2012). *Depression: A Public Feeling*. Durham, NC: Duke University Press.

Davies, J. (2012). *The Importance of Suffering: The Value and Meaning of Emotional Discontent*. London, New York: Routledge.

De Graeve, K. (2015). Geographies of migration and relatedness: Transmigrancy in open transnational adoptive parenting. *Social & Cultural Geography*, 16(5), pp. 522–535.

Deleuze, G. & Guattari, F. (1987). *A Thousand Plateaus: Capitalism and Schizophrenia*. Minneapolis, MN: University of Minnesota Press.

Dragojlovic, A. (2011). 'Did you Know my Father?': The zone of unspeakability as postcolonial legacy. *Australian Feminist Studies*, 69(26), pp. 317–332.

Dragojlovic, A. (2014). The search for sensuous geographies of absence: Indisch mediation of loss. *Bijdragen tot de Taal-, Land- en Volkenkunde* (*Journal of the Humanities and Social Sciences of Southeast Asia*), 170(4), pp. 473–503.

Dragojlovic, A. (2015a). Hunted by miscegenation: gender, the white Australian policy and the construction of Indisch family narratives. *Journal of Intercultural Studies*, 36(1), pp. 54–70.

Dragojlovic, A. (2015b). Affective geographies: Intergenerational hauntings, bodily affectivity and multiracial subjectivities. *Subjectivity*, 8, pp. 315–334.

Dragojlovic, A. (2016a). *Beyond Bali: Subaltern Citizens and Post-Colonial Intimacy*. Amsterdam: Amsterdam University Press.

Dragojlovic, A. (2016b). Playing family: Unruly relationality, and transnational motherhood. *Gender, Place and Culture: Journal of Feminist Geography*, 23(2), pp. 243–256.

Essed, P. (1991). *Understanding Everyday Racism: An Interdisciplinary Theory*. Newbury Park: Sage.

Essed, P. & Hoving, I., eds. (2014). *Dutch Racism*. Amsterdam: Rodopi.

Essed, P. & Hoving, I. (2014 Innocence, smug ignorance, resentment: An introduction to Dutch racism. In Essed, P. and Hoving, I., eds, *Dutch Racism*. Amsterdam: Rodopi, pp. 9–30.

Goldberg, D. T. (1993). *Racist Culture: Philosophy and the Politics of Meaning*. Cambridge: Blackwell.

Halberstam, J. J. (2011). *The Queer Art of Failure*. Durham, NC: Duke University Press.

Herman, E. (2008). *Kinship by Design: A History of Adoption in the Modern United States*. Chicago: University of Chicago Press.

Hjern, A., Lindblad, F. & Vinnerljung, B. (2002). Suicide, psychiatric illness, and social maladjustment in intercountry adoptees in Sweden: A cohort study. *The Lancet*, 360(9331), pp. 443–448.

Hoksbergen, R. (2011). *Kinderen die niet konden blijven. Zestig jaar adoptie in Nederland*. Soesterberg: Aspekt.

Howell, S. (2003). Kinning: The creation of life trajectories in transnational adoptive families. *Journal of the Royal Anthropological Institute*, 9, pp. 465–484.

Howell, S. (2009). Adoption of the unrelated child: Some challenges to the anthropological study of kinship. *Annual Review of Anthropology*, 38, pp. 149–166.

Hübinette, T. (2004). A critique of intercountry adoption. In Dudley, W., ed., *Issues in Adoption: Current Controversies*. Farmington Hills: Greenhaven Press, pp. 66–71.

Hübinette, T. (2007). Disembedded and free-floating bodies out-of-place and out-of-control: examining the borderline existence of adopted Koreans. *Adoption & Culture: The Interdisciplinary Journal of the Alliance for the Study of Adoption and Culture*, 1(1), pp. 129–162.

Hübinette, T. & Tigervall, C. (2009). To be non-white in a colour-blind society: Conversations with adoptees and adoptive parents in Sweden on everyday racism. *Journal of Intercultural Studies*, 30(4), pp. 335–353.

Illouz, E. (2008). *Saving the Modern Soul: Therapy, Emotions, and the Culture of Self-Help*. Berkeley, CA: University of California Press.

Jacobson, H. (2008). *Culture Keeping: White Mothers, International Adoption, and the Negotiation of Family Difference*. Nashville, TN: Vanderbilt University Press.

Johansson-Kark, M. I., Rasmussen, F. & Hjern, A. (2002). Overweight among international adoptees in Sweden: a population-based study. *Acta Paediatrica*, 91(7), pp. 827–832.

Kawash, S. (2011). New directions in motherhood studies. *Signs*, 36(4), pp. 969–1003.

Kim, J. E. (2010). *Adopted Territory: Transnational Korean Adoptees and the Politics of Belonging*. Durham, NC: Duke University Press.

Knudsen, B. T. & Stage, C. (2015). Introduction: Affective methodologies. In Knudsen, B. T. & Stage, C., eds, *Affective Methodologies*. UK: Palgrave Macmillan, pp. 1–22.

Leinaweaver, J. & van Wichelen, S. (2015). The geography of transnational adoption: Kin and place in globalization. *Social & Cultural Geography*, 16(5), pp. 499–507.

Leys, R. (2011a) The turn to affect: A critique. *Critical Inquiry*, 37(3), pp. 434–472.

Leys, R. (2011b). Affect and intention: A reply to William E. Connolly. *Critical Inquiry*, 37(3), pp. 799–805.

Lindblad, F., Hjern, A. & Vinnerljung, B. (2003). Intercountry adopted children as young adults a Swedish cohort study. *American Journal of Orthopsychiatry*, 73(2), pp. 190–202.

Love, H. (2007). *Feeling Backward: Loss and the Politics of Queer History*. Cambridge, MA: Harvard University Press.

Lucassen, J. & Penninx, R. (1993). *Nieuwkomers, Nakomelingen, Nederlanders: Immigranten in Nederland 1550–1993*. Amsterdam: Het Spinhuis.

108   *Suffering, the lived body and mobility*

Marre, D. (2007). I want her to learn her language and maintain her culture: Transnational adoptive families' views of 'cultural origins'. In Wade, P., ed., *Race, Ethnicity and Nation: Perspectives from Kinship and Genetics*. New York, NY: Berghahn Books, pp. 73–93.

Massumi, B. (2002). *Parables for the Virtual: Movement, Affect, Sensation*. Durham, NC: Duke University Press.

Mol, A. (2002). *The Body Multiple: Ontology in Medical Practice*. Durham, NC: Duke University Press.

Navaro-Yashin, Y. (2012). *The Make-Believe Space: Affective Geography in a Postwar Polity*. Durham, NC: Duke University Press.

Razack, S. (2002). *When Place Becomes Race. Race, Space, and the Law: Unmapping a White Settler Society*. Toronto: Between the Lines.

Rose, N. (1990). *Governing the Soul: The Shaping of the Private Self*. London, New York: Routledge.

Sedgwick, E. K. (1993). *Tendencies*. Durham, NC: Duke University Press.

Seidman, S. (2004). *Beyond the Closet: The Transformation of Gay and Lesbian Life*. London, New York: Routledge.

Seigworth, G. (2003). *Fashioning a Stave, or, Singing Life*. In Slack, J. D., ed., *Animations of Deleuze and Guattari*. New York: Peter Lang, pp. 75–105.

Selman, P. (2002). Intercountry adoption in the new millennium; the 'quiet migration' revisited. *Population Research and Policy Review*, 21(3), pp. 205–225.

Thelen, T. (2015). Care as social organization: Creating, maintaining and dissolving significant relations. *Anthropological Theory*, 5(4), pp. 497–515.

Thrift, N. (2008). *Non-Representational Theory: Space, Politics, Affect*. New York: Routledge.

Tieman, W. (2006). *Mental Health in Young Adult Intercountry Adoptees*. Rotterdam: Optima Grafische Commuicatie.

Van Amersfoort, H. & Van Niekerk, M. (2006). Immigration as a colonial inheritance: Post-colonial immigrants in the Netherlands, 1945–2002. *Journal of Ethnic and Migration Studies*, 32(2), pp. 323–346.

Van Wichelen, S. (2014). Medicine as moral technology: somatic economies and the making up of adoptees. *Medical Anthropology*, 33, pp. 109–127.

Van Wichelen, S. (2015). Scales of grievability: On moving children and the geopolitics of precariousness. *Social & Cultural Geography*, 16(5), pp. 552–566.

Volkman, T. A. (2003). Embodying Chinese culture: Transnational adoption in North America. *Social Text*, 21, pp. 29–55.

Volkman, T. A., ed. (2005). *Cultures of Transnational Adoption*. Durham, NC: Duke University Press.

von Borczyskowski, A., Hjern, A. Lindblad, F. and B. Vinnerljung (2006). Suicidal behaviour in national and international adult adoptees: A Swedish cohort study. *Social Psychiatry and Psychiatric Epidemiology*, 41(2), pp. 95–102.

Walton, J. (2015). Feeling it: Understanding Korean adoptees' experiences of embodied identity. *Journal of Intercultural Studies*, 36(4), pp. 395–412.

Watson, N., McKie, L., Hughes, B. & Gregory, S. (2004). (Inter)dependence, needs and care: The potential for disability and feminist theorists to develop an emancipatory model. *Sociology*, 38(2), pp. 331–350.

Wekker, G. (2016). *White Innocence: Paradoxes of Colonialism and Race*. Durham, NC: Duke University Press.

Williams, F. (2001). In and beyond New Labour: Towards a new political ethics of care. *Critical Social Policy*, 21(4), pp. 467–493.

Willing, I. (2006). Beyond the Vietnam War adoptions: Representing our transracial lives. In Trenka, J., Oparah, C. & Shin, S. Y. eds, *Outsiders Within: Racial Crossings and Adoption Politics*. Cambridge, MA: South End Press, pp. 275–285.

Willing, I. (2009). The celebrity adoptions phenomenon: Emerging critiques from 'ordinary' adoptive parents. In Spark, C. & Cuthbert, D. eds, *Other People's Children: Adoption in Australia*. Melbourne: Australian Scholarly Publishing, pp. 241–256.

Yngvesson, B. (2010). *Belonging in an Adopted World*. Chicago: University of Chicago Press.

Yngvesson, B. (2012). Transnational adoption and European immigration politics: Producing the national body in Sweden. *Indiana Journal of Global Legal Studies*, 19, pp. 327–345.

Part 3

Sites of care, self-help and coping with suffering

5 The practice of radical affectivity
Evoking suffering as a healing modality

In this chapter, we argue that in addressing and reconfiguring suffering, attention must be paid to how negative affect might be evoked as a healing modality. We focus our analytical lens on how negative affect can be reclaimed rather than repressed, and explore what kinds of ontological transformations this might offer. Thus, we analyse how engaging with suffering as unhappy forms of affect can be both the solution to and the site of suffering, concurrently. We focus on how a group healing method – Family Constellation Therapy (FCT) – seeks to heal its subjects' senses of suffering and trauma by intentionally intervening into its participants' pre-cognitive and pre-subjective states. FCT does so by creating an atmosphere of suffering that is expected to provoke negative feelings such as unhappiness, shame, depression, failure, anxiety, low self-esteem, suicidal tendencies, rage and self-harm.

We analyse an FCT session organised for adult adoptees by support group *For Adoptees* in Amsterdam,[1] the Netherlands. Unlike the discussion sessions that *For Adoptees* also organises, and which were discussed in Chapter 4, the FCT sessions that *For Adoptees* organises are mostly concerned with interpersonal relationships between biological and adopted family members, as well as intimate relationships. This is not to say that racialisation and othering do not play important roles in interpersonal relationships. In FCT sessions in general, attendees re-enact situations that are sites of grief, loss and conflict by 'meeting' and 'interacting' with other participants who, for the purpose of the re-enacted situations, stand in the place of their birth and adopted parents, siblings who passed away, or family members with whom they have ongoing, seemingly unresolvable problems. Through these sessions, *For Adoptees* attendees intentionally engage with negative emotions in order to seek opportunities that may lead to possibilities of self-transformation – in this case, an ambiguous sense of self-sovereignty[2] that is autonomous from the attendees' everyday experiences of negative feelings and related suffering (see also Chapter 4), and yet inexorably linked to it and invested in continuity within negativity.

The ethnographic material that we analyse here was collected by Dragojlovic in 2013–2014 through participant observation at numerous FCT group sessions, as well as in open-ended interviews with participants after the sessions, including immediately after the sessions but also months and years later. The material

urges us to employ an analytic approach from the scholarly literature that problematises the understanding of the human body as a singular, bounded entity
(Blackman, 2008, 2012; Latour, 2004; Mol, 2002), and to pay attention to how
affective assemblages of suffering operate through and across the binary oppositions of cognitive and affective, intentional and non-intentional. Our discussion in
this chapter furthers the argument that we make in the book as a whole; namely,
that caring relations need to be approached as multifaceted and, in the case of
healing modality (FCT) discussed here, understood through intersubjective and
intercorporeal experiences of suffering. In what follows, we first provide a background for the analysis of the ethnographic material by providing an overview of
FCT. Second, inspired by 'negative turn' in the queer and feminist scholarship
that emphasises the productive potentials of negative feelings and negative states
of being (Ahmed, 2010; Blackman, 2015; Cvetkovich, 2012; Halberstam, 2011;
Love, 2007) we analyse how the practice of what we call 'radical affectivity' is
evoked, performed and given meaning at the FCT sessions, which insist on pro-
voking emotional suffering as a way of achieving self-transformation. Finally,
it is important to stress that we do not aim to make claims about the efficacy of
FCT, but rather to ethnographically explore how such therapy is approached as an
avenue to individual and group empowerment while seeing emotional distress as a
process that occurs intercorporeally, and the human body as relational and always
in a process of becoming.

Family Constellation Therapy: the approach

FCT is an alternative therapeutic method developed by German psychotherapist
Bert Hellinger in the 1980s. This method offers somatic therapy and is a brief,
solution-focused experiential method that is based on family systems therapy,
existential phenomenology, and the ancestral reverence of the Zulu people of
South Africa, wherein ancestors are perceived as having an active presence in the
everyday lives of their descendants (Cohen, 2006). While such an understanding
about ancestral presence exists among many different cultures around the world,
Hellinger (who lived as a Christian missionary in South Africa before becoming
a psychotherapist) has interpreted the belief as being something unique to Zulu
people (Hellinger et al., 1998). The FCT process has also been influenced by
'psychodrama', developed by Jacob Moreno (1945) as a form of psychotherapy,
and by family sculptures, developed by psychiatrists Iván Böszörményi-Nagy and
Geraldine Spark (1973). What FCT retains from these approaches is a focus on
the client's personal issues, and the selection of other attendees to stand in as representatives of members of the client's family system.

FCT group sessions generally consist of one facilitator (sometimes assisted by
two or three colleagues), and between ten and thirty attendees. Those attending
can have a specific question that they would like to work on and seek resolution
for, or they can attend solely in order to stand as representatives. Many of Dragojlovic's interlocutors initially attended the sessions not to ask specific questions
for themselves, but rather to have a better understanding of how FCT operates,

hoping that their participation would help them to decide whether they wanted to use it as a therapeutic method for the resolution of their own issues. The sessions are usually held in a closed space such as a room hired for the occasion or in the home of the facilitator, and the participants usually begin by sitting around the room. When the first attendee asks his or her question and selects other attendees to be representatives to stand for his or her family members, the representatives move into the centre of the room and are expected to be 'able to tune into the unconscious, collective will of the family system' of the client asking the question (Cohen, 2006, p. 226). Cohen (2006) argues that, according to Böszörményi-Nagy and Spark (1973), this is an unexplainable mechanism that influences individual behaviour within the family system. This mechanism has been also referred to by FCT practitioners as 'the knowing field', after Rupert Sheldrake's (1995) morphic resonance. Relying on the power of 'the knowing field', the facilitator positions representatives in a certain order, and then waits to see what kinds of movements will spontaneously develop between them. The facilitator asks representatives how they feel in certain positions, and about the direction within the field in which they would like to move. Responding to responses from the representatives and their personal understandings of what the right movement should be, the facilitator experimentally moves the representatives within the field. Looking for harmonious movement (for example, if two representatives who represent people in the family system who had previously had a conflict are content looking at each other), the facilitator makes healing statements (for example, about forgiveness), which the representatives then repeat. Cohen writes that:

> [the r]epresentation of the ancestral field literally manifests a new point of view. These are not dictated or scripted by the facilitator, nor are they expressions of the client's inner dialogue or emotion . . . they appear to emerge spontaneously from the constellation itself . . . as if the ancestral field, Böszörményi-Nagy's mechanism, has a mind, a message of its own and, now, a forum for expression. The ancestors' representatives become characters in a living novella, altering the meaning of past events and reconfiguring the family system.
>
> (Cohen, 2006, p. 229)

The client is expected to integrate the image of the healing over time and is not expected to talk about what happened at the constellation to others or to try to consciously remember it. The client is instead encouraged to 'forget' the details of the events that occurred at the session with the explanation by the facilitator that what happened 'works on the unconscious level'. Sometimes, the unconscious level is also interpreted as a level of the family soul. While dynamics at the constellation sessions vary, most of the facilitators agree that the healing from the session will benefit not only the client, but also people in client's family system even if they do not know that the client conducted the healing.

While based in the psychotherapeutic tradition, FCT differentiates from conventional psychotherapy in several important ways. First, the client speaks only rarely, and second, the primary aim of the therapy is to 'identify and release pre-reflexive transgenerational patterns embedded within the family system, not to explore or process narrative, cognitive, or emotional content' (Cohen, 2006, p. 226). Over the years, this approach has expanded from group sessions to include individual sessions and constellation workshops for businesses and organisations. The constellation workshops claim to assist the resolution of interpersonal conflicts within organisations, and to assist the development better interpersonal communication between workers in order to enhance productivity and effectiveness.

Method

The research on FCT practices presented in this chapter was gathered as part of a subfield of Dragojlovic's ethnographic research on memory and genealogy work conducted in the Netherlands. During her ethnographic research, Dragojlovic attended and participated in numerous group therapy sessions and worked closely with five practitioners and their clients. All of the practitioners combined this method with other therapeutic methods, such as psychotherapy, integrative therapy and art therapy. Two of the practitioners worked as social workers, while for the other three, therapy work was their main profession. During this period, Dragojlovic also attended training workshops for existing and future therapists in 'systemic work'. The latter term is preferred by Dragojlovic's interlocutors as it enables them to work with groups, individuals and in institutional settings. Thus, the training sessions usually aimed to cover many different modes and settings for 'systemic work'. Almost without exception, all the clients that took part in the sessions that formed part of Dragojlovic's research were involved in various other forms of alternative health practices in addition to FCT. These practices included alternative food consumption, yoga, art and exercise therapy, reiki, acupuncture, quantum therapy, ayahuasca consumption and different neo-shamanic rituals. Additionally, most of the clients had trained (or were training while participating in FCT) as psychologists, psychiatrists, psychoanalysts, integrative therapists, social workers, acupuncturists, art therapists, or other similar professions. Some of the clients were taking prescribed antidepressants, while some used to take them but had given up. In addition, several of the clients were regular consumers of so-called 'soft drugs' (those that are legal in the Netherlands, such as marijuana). The facilitators who took part in the research perceived FCT as being exceptionally suitable for adoptees in particular, who seemed to hold unresolved grief for or in connection with their biological parents. At the same time, FCT sessions with adoptees were seen by facilitators as more challenging than others, as adoptees have 'two families in their systems: biological and adopted'.

The ethnographic case study: what is wrong with suffering?

In Chapter 4, we observed that the leadership of the *For Adoptees* support group continually stressed the importance of emotional suffering as an integral part of what it means to be a human, rather than as a psychiatric problem that requires medicalisation and antidepressant therapy. The coordinators of *For Adoptees* did not see suffering as an emotion to be avoided or chemically altered, but rather something to be self-reflectively engaged with. Such an approach in many ways echoes the work of British anthropologist and psychotherapist James Davies (2012), who argues for the potential value of suffering in personal, social and clinical settings. As we demonstrated in Chapter 4, the *For Adoptees* group meetings were concerned with reconceptualising strong emotions such as rage, shame, a sense of unworthiness, guilt, abandonment, a chronic feeling of loss as things that are related to the broader cultural, and social context in which a person's life is situated, rather than as solely belonging to an individual adoptee. FCT practitioners contend that the human bodies are containers of truth that often cannot be verbally articulated; in order to reach that truth, one requires what was referred to as 'digging deeper', through an intersubjective healing process. This meant exploring the pre-reflexive and pre-cognitive, and what lay outside of their self-reflexive narration. While FCT does not in itself postulate the importance of suffering, group sessions are meant to bring about affective states capable of making visible (through bodily movements) and articulable the emotional distress that is located in the participants' bodies, which is otherwise perceived to exist outside of the participants' cognitive knowledge and articulation. The experiences of dying and survivorship discussed in Chapter 6 may involve similar dynamics. This understanding of the body is somewhat resonant with the argument made by American somatic psychologist Stanley Keleman, who said that '[t]he body cannot lie. It is incapable of lying' (1981, p. 66). While for Keleman (1981, 1985) and his followers, the body is understood as embodying emotional experiences, being patterned by them, and being repositories of dark secrets, the FCT practitioners with whom Dragojlovic conducted her ethnographic research perceived this bodily capacity as an intergenerational process. In other words, the individual human body is perceived as a repository of ancestral habits, secrets and traumas several generations removed.[3] Here, bodies are treated as 'lived bodies', with the capacity to affect and be affected, and always in a process of becoming. This approach resonates closely with scholarly arguments that criticise the understanding of the human body as a static, singular, bounded entity (Blackman, 2008, 2012; Csordas, 2008; Latour, 2004; Mol, 2002).

The FCT session analysed here took place on Saturday, 22 March, 2014 in The Hague. The session was facilitated by Henk, who had been a member of *For Adoptees* since its establishment. Beginning in 2011, Henk has run regular FCT sessions (usually every two to three months) specifically designed for the participation of adult adoptees. Like some other facilitators, Henk also conducts group sessions for non-adoptees, and frequently assists Indisch (Indo-Dutch) facilitators working on FCT sessions dedicated to Indisch issues. This collaboration between Indisch and adoptee facilitators is both interesting and important. Indisch people trace their family heritage to the intergenerational, interracial and intercultural mixing of Indonesian women and Dutch (or other European) men and/or of

Indisch people themselves in the colonial Dutch East Indies, which existed from 1600 to 1942. After the end of the Second World War (1945) and Indonesian independence (internationally recognised in 1949), Indisch people, being Dutch citizens, moved from Indonesia to, for the most part, the Netherlands, Australia, the United States and Canada. Both Indisch and adoptee FCT facilitators share a common interest in uncovering deep-seated, contested senses of being different, of not completely belonging to Dutch society, and of being related to 'elusive elsewheres' (Dragojlovic, 2014). As we argued in Chapters 3 and 4, and as Dragojlovic has argued elsewhere (Dragojlovic, 2016), such feelings are related to a complex matrix of mobility, historical violence and experiences of everyday racism in Dutch society. Feeling a profound connection to the geographies in which most of them had never been, Indisch people and transnational adoptees share a common interest in understanding these connections. As such, many of them have trained to become facilitators in FCT at courses organised specifically for them. Henk trained at such a course during 2009 and 2010, and made strong working relations with several Indisch people, with whom he now often facilitates FCT sessions on a joint basis.

In the above-mentioned session for adult adoptees, Henk was assisted by Marla, an Indisch woman who had undergone her training at the same time as him. These two were accompanied by Andreas,[4] an Indisch country musician who has dedicated several of his solo albums to Indisch themes, particularly as they relate to a sense of loss, suffering, historical violence and parental suffering, and thus serve as a specific form of Indisch memory and genealogy work. Andreas is frequently invited by facilitators to participate at FCT sessions that are focused on Indisch people, adoptees or a mix of the two, in order to help participants 'tune into their family fields' with his lyrics (as explained by facilitators). All of the facilitators who participated in the research presented in this chapter unanimously agreed that the FCT method was specifically well-suited to treating problems related to grief and separation, and as such, specifically suited to the examination of the loss of biological family that all adoptees have suffered.

In the FCT group workshops Dragojlovic attended, the facilitator would open the session by taking a genealogical chart of each of the participants, often by drawing them on large sheets of paper attached to a whiteboard and dedicating a page to each participant. During the sessions, these drawings would be used to help the facilitator position the representatives, as well as, at the end of the sessions, to help the participants discuss the dynamics that were experienced at the sessions and their resolutions. While drawing the genealogy chart, facilitators would often pose questions such as, 'how are you going in your life?', 'how did it go with your adoptive parents?', 'what is the special issue you would like to work on?' This, together with the 'healing' part of the session, would usually last between 30 and 50 minutes per client. Some facilitators spend as long as 2 or 3 hours on an individual client, while others insist on swift movements designed to prevent the representatives from 'thinking', and rather force them to be in the flow of pre-reflexive, pre-cognitive states that, it is believed, will be animated in the 'knowing field'. The sessions facilitated by Henk utilised the swift method.

Twenty-five people attended the FCT session in The Hague, having travelled from different parts of the country for the occasion. The participants gathered at 9 am, at a venue hired from the local municipality for the occasion, and were offered tea and coffee refreshments on their arrival. By 10 am, all the participants were seated on comfortable cushions on the floor in a circle around Henk, who was seated on a chair. Andrea and Marla, who were assisting Henk in the session, were seated on the floor on his right and left side respectively. The participants were made up of 11 men and 14 women, aged between 18 and 49. The participants were given minimal information about how the session would proceed, and no consent form was sought.

Prior to the commencement of the session, Henk had told Dragojlovic that four of the participants in attendance that day were regular clients of his (that is, he was their personal/life coach), three were regular attendees of *For Adoptees* group meetings but had not attended an FCT session before, while he had never had any interaction with the rest of them. Henk opened the session by welcoming the participants and inviting everybody to close their eyes for a short meditation. This meditation was designed to help the group 'tune easily into the knowing field', as he put it. Following this, Henk invited all participants to introduce themselves by name, the country from which they had been adopted, if they wanted to have their case constellated, and the reasons why they were attending. Henk specifically stressed that these introductions should be brief, because 'the less we know about each other, the better results we will get from the constellation.' Most of the participants said they were attending as they wished to learn more about 'adoptees condition', and to understand themselves better. Only seven people of the 25 participants had never attended an FCT session before. The others had attended sessions before, but only as representatives or observers, or had had their questions constellated already, and perceived the current session as a way to learn more about the process.

Through her research, Dragojlovic learned that many attendees go to different facilitators, searching to find the one who will be best suited for the resolution of their particular problems. The most common way of describing how the right facilitator had been found was, 'you know it in your body when a solution is found . . . You feel lighter; better. You see that your everyday life is changing for the better.' The facilitating style of facilitators can vary greatly, and many facilitators told me about the numerous strategies they had implemented to seek to 'brand' their own approach. Some were more interested in combining what they do with 'traditional shamanism'. This practice is often seen in facilitators who have Indonesian or Korean backgrounds and who, on the way to their own self-discovery, found shamanistic ancestry. Other facilitators were more keen in looking for 'scientific proof' that the FCT method can be applied to various settings – from intergenerational issues to interpersonal communication in the workplace, and the increase of productivity in large corporations. As Henk insisted on constellating as many questions as possible, 14 separate questions were enacted during the session that took place on 22 March, 2014. We offer a detailed ethnographic description of three constellations that took place on the day, which addressed different aspects of the adoptees' lives. The focus here is on how an affective atmosphere is evoked, managed, given meaning and used as a healing process.

Annelies

Annelies was among the first participants to raise her hand to have her question constellated. Adopted from Korea, she appeared to be in her 30s, and looked fragile and insecure while speaking in front of the group. None of the particularities of her life were known to the group, but Annelies said her main problem had always been a strong sense of loneliness and insecurity, and a feeling that she had no stable ground on which to stand. Henk asked her if she wanted to choose a representative for herself first. Annelies looked carefully around the room, approached another woman who had herself been adopted from Korea and who, in body shape and height, somewhat resembled Annelies, and asked her, 'Would you represent me?' Annelies then extended her right hand to the woman for a handshake, as instructed by the facilitator. Once the woman accepted Annelies's hand, she was led to the centre of the room. Henk then asked Annelies whether she wanted to choose a representative for her biological mother, at which she looked at him with a heightened sense of fear and anxiety. Annelies lowered her gaze and shook her head, but did not speak. Henk proceeded to choose a representative of the biological mother on Annelies's behalf, asking Annelies in a soft voice to help him by approving his choice. She approved the first person he suggested by nodding her head, then started to sob. Henk asked both representatives (for Annelies and for the biological mother) to keep their eyes closed and led the 'mother' in front of the 'daughter', leaving about two metres' distance between them, He said, 'Annelies, open your eyes, this is your birth mother standing in front of you.' The representative opened her eyes, not expressing any emotions, and just stared at the 'mother', who was then also asked to open her eyes by the words, 'Birth mother of Anneliese, your daughter is standing in front of you.' The 'mother' looked at the 'daughter', who still had an expressionless face, and quickly, as if frightened, turned her body away from the 'daughter', and fixated her gaze on the floor. Henk asked the mother, 'Can you look at your daughter?' 'No!' replied the woman briskly, continuing to stare at the ground. He then turned to the 'daughter', who was still staring at the 'mother'. He asked her, 'How are you feeling, Annelies?' The representative for Annelies replied, 'I do not feel anything.' The real Annelies was carefully monitoring the scene, tears rolling down her face.

Henk proceeded by saying, 'We might have not chosen the best representative for Anneliese. It might be better if Annelies stands for herself.' Henk thanked the representative, asked Annelies to close her eyes, and led her to the place where the representative had been standing. He said, 'Annelies, open your eyes. Your birth mother is in front of you.' Opening her eyes, Annelies looked at her 'mother', who was still staring at the ground. Annelies' body began to shake as if she would fall over. Henk, who was standing next to her, took her by the arm, softly saying 'easy, easy', and then instructed her to say, 'Birth mother, I am here.' Expending what seemed like exceptional effort, Anneliese repeated his words, fighting for breath after each word. The 'mother', however, did not move, and did not look at her 'daughter'. At this point, Henk signalled to his assistant. Marla chose a representative from the group of people sitting in the circle and asked her to lie on the floor where the 'mother' was staring. In response to this, the 'mother' leaned towards the person laying on the ground. Henk asked the 'mother', 'How are you feeling, birth mother?' The 'mother' remained speechless, and kept staring at the person on the ground. Marla and Henk exchanged glances, and Marla chose another representative, and instructed them to lie on the floor next to the first representative. Seeing that the 'mother' leaned even further towards the people on the ground, Henk said, 'Birth mother, you have another child who is alive and she is here.' The 'mother' quickly said, 'leave me alone'. At these words, Annelies almost collapsed, as if she had been stabbed in her stomach with a sharp object. She sobbed inconsolably and Henk struggled to keep her in the standing position. Marla took hold of Annelies and whispered what seemed like soothing words to her, while Henk attempted to divert the attention of the 'mother' away from the people on the floor, to no avail.

Eventually, Henk thanked the 'mother' and the representative returned to sit on the floor among the other observers. Henk explained, 'Annelies, your birth mother is suffering a deep trauma. She is completely fixated on her two other children who died that she cannot see anything else. We all need to know that some of our mothers gave us up because they had too much pain in their lives, and no one to help them.' By this time, most of the participants sitting about the room were crying. Two of them who had been overwhelmed by their emotions left the room, sobbing loudly. At this point, Henk decided to call on 'Korean mothers', inviting one by one the women from the group who had been sitting on the floor to get up and stand behind Annelies. Henk asked the women – some 10 of them – to place their hands on Annelies's shoulder. In the meantime, Annelies, who was still being held by Marla, became a bit calmer and confirmed this verbally when asked how she was feeling by the facilitator. Henk explained that adoptees are not only supported by mothers from the nations in which they were born, but also by fathers and by other people. He then called on the other participants to stand as 'fathers' and these other 'people'. Together with the 'mothers', the group made a long line of people standing behind Annelies. 'How are you feeling now?' Henk asked Annelies. In a soft voice, she replied, 'A bit better.' Henk asked everyone standing in the line to close their eyes and to send all the energy they could from Korean mothers, fathers and other people to Annelies. After several minutes spent in silence, the constellation was dismantled.

Nadia

One of the other participants who had her system constellated at Henk's FCT session was Nadia, a woman in her late 40s who had been adopted from Sri Lanka. Nadia did not want to have a representative for herself, as she had done this at a previous constellation session and was not satisfied with the results. She came to the session wishing to reconnect with her biological father, who she knew had been an enemy soldier. While Nadia wanted to tell the group more about him, Henk interrupted her, saying, 'we do not need to hear it from you. Let the field guide us towards the resolution.' Henk then asked Nadia to choose a representative each for her biological and adopted mothers, instructing Nadia and the two 'mothers' to stand in the middle, making a triangle. When Henk asked them all to open their eyes and look wherever felt most comfortable, both of the 'mothers' looked at Nadia. Nadia first faced her 'birth mother', and then turned and looked at her 'adopted mother'. Asked how she felt by the facilitator, Nadia said, 'good. I am fine looking at my birth mother, but I feel closer to my adopted mother.' When Henk asked her to choose a representative for her adopted father, Nadia loudly exclaimed, 'Noooo!', and began to run around the room, almost stepping on the other participants who were still sitting on the floor. Henk tried to calm her down, but Nadia began to scream even louder and to run faster, saying, 'leave me alone, leave me alone . . .' For a moment, Henk stopped and Marla approached Nadia, but Marla too struggled to get a hold of her. Next, Henk yelled loudly, 'Nadia, your adopted father is not here. Snap out of it!' Hearing these words and being comforted by Marla, Nadia stopped running and screaming. Still visibly shaken, she returned to the position she had been standing in previously.

The atmosphere in the room was tense. Some of the participants who had stood up while Nadia was running around the room returned to their sitting positions, while others fidgeted nervously and whispered among each other. Henk invited all participants to close their eyes, take a deep breath and take a couple of minutes to meditate. Some minutes later, his voice invited all those present to open their eyes, and asked Nadia if she wanted to choose a representative for her biological father. With a smile and a sense of excitement on her face, Nadia chose the oldest man from the group and then returned to the position she had been standing in. The 'biological father' stood up next to Henk and was then led to stand next to Nadia's 'biological mother'. As soon as the man stood next to her, the woman jumped away and turned her back to him, while he was facing her. Asked by Henk how he felt, the 'biological father' said, 'Lonely, abandoned . . .' Henk asked him to face Nadia's 'adopted mother'. The 'biological father' and 'adopted mother' looked at each other with a sense of sympathy, and the facilitator asked the 'biological father' to tell the 'adopted mother', 'Thank you for taking care of my daughter.' After this, the 'adopted mother' was thanked for her participation and asked to re-join the observers.

When her 'biological mother' turned her back on the 'biological father', Nadia began sobbing, and by the time the 'adopted mother' sat back down, Nadia's body was shaking ferociously. Henk made various attempts to get the 'biological mother' and the 'biological father' to communicate with one another, but the 'biological mother' refused to engage with the 'biological father'. Henk thanked the 'biological mother' for taking part in Nadia's constellation and she sat down. Henk explained that, despite our wishes for our biological parents to have good communication, this is not always possible. He turned to Nadia, who was still sobbing and being comforted by Marla, and then to the 'biological father', who was still looking in direction of where Nadia's 'biological mother' had been standing. Henk told him, 'Amal [the name of Nadia's biological father], your daughter Nadia is here.' The man moved suddenly and began looking at Nadia, which made him smile. The facilitator asked him to say, 'Nadia, you are my daughter and I love you.' His voice was imbued with feelings of love, as was the expression of kindness on his face. Nadia jumped, hugged the man and stated repeatedly, 'I love you, daddy.' The two stayed in the hug for a very long time before Henk decided to separate them. Seeing the resistance on Nadia's part, he asked her to tell the man, 'You will always be my father', and asked him to tell Nadia, 'You will always be my daughter.' With this, the constellation ended. This session was the last before our lunch break and at the end, Nadia approached the man who had represented her biological father, thanked him and continued to have a conversation with him.

When the session resumed after the break, Henk announced that Andreas would be performing some of his songs. Andreas' songs were dedicated, first, to his parents (who had suffered during the Pacific War), second, to Indisch descendants (who live as migrants in the Netherlands and other parts of the world), and third to adoptees, most of whose ancestors had lived through the brutal wars in Korea and Sri Lanka. During the performance, Andreas and many people in the audience became tearful. During the song entitled 'To my lost father', the atmosphere in the room erupted. Many of the people in the room began to sob loudly. Halfway through the song, Nadia jumped from her seated position and began screaming, 'Daddy, don't leave me!' She fiercely hugged the man who was represented her biological father during her constellation. The man seemed shocked by Nadia's expression of affection and pushed her away, which brought about an outburst from Nadia, accompanied by screams, sobbing and not wanting to let go of the man. Henk, Marla and Andreas pulled Nadia away from the man, leading her out of the room and tried to calm her down with words and a glass of water. The other participants began to leave the room. One of them stated that an ambulance should be called; that Nadia needed medical help. For about 30 minutes, the place was in a state of commotion. Some people said that they would never ask their own questions, that the 'method is very dangerous', and that they were 'feeling sick of their own and other people's pain'. After calming down somewhat, Nadia called for her son to come and pick her up. Five other participants excused themselves and left the session. After an early afternoon tea break, those who had stayed reconvened for the final part of the session.

Some days later, when Henk and Dragojlovic were discussing the particularities of Nadia's session, Henk told Dragojlovic that Nadia had been his client for 10 months at that point. Henk knew that Nadia's adopted father had sexually molested her, and this was the reason for her adopted parents' divorce. Based on this knowledge, Henk presumed that it was very important for Nadia to reconnect with her adopted father during the constellation. He continued, 'in this case, there is so much pain that the best way to deal with it is to be re-traumatised in a supportive environment (i.e. at the constellation), surrounded by other adoptees. She needs to have witnesses to what happened to her. If she was able to face her adopted father in the constellation, that would take power away from him outside of these sessions, and she would feel safe and strong.' Despite Nadia's behaviour, Henk maintained that the session was helpful for her, but perhaps not enough. He suggested that she would need more time to 'integrate everything', and should undertake another constellation session in the future, when 'she feels strong enough to face her adopted father in another constellation'.

Marcel

Marcel was a man in his late 30s who had been adopted from Haiti and who wanted to 'see his current family dynamic in a constellation'. He was having problems with his wife and, assuming that these problems might be related to his adoption, wanted to 'test it'. When asked to choose a representative for his wife, Marcel chose a woman of around his age with long blonde hair, who had been adopted from Russia. We learned later that the representative looked quite similar to his Dutch wife. To represent himself, he chose an Afro-Brazilian man. Walking into the circle, the 'wife' was asked by the facilitator to repeat that she is now Elsa, which she did. When the man who was representing Marcel was brought to stand next to 'Elsa', she immediately turned away from him and ran to the exit door. Speaking softly, Henk invited two people to stand as representatives of Marcel and Elsa's two children, and then in a louder voice said to 'Elsa', who was facing away, 'Elsa, your children are here.' On hearing this, 'Elsa' quickly came back, looking at her 'children' with a smile. Marcel's representative was standing out of her eyesight.

The facilitator then invited three men to stand next to Marcel and represent his father and three brothers, who the facilitator knew lived in Haiti. He then asked 'Elsa' if she could look at 'Marcel'. Very slowly, with a sense of fear and anticipation, she turned her head towards him and said, 'I can, as long as he is far away from me and the children.' Henk interpreted that to mean that Marcel's white Dutch wife found him to be a weak man and disliked him for that, but that now, when he was supported by his male kin from Haiti, she had a better opinion of him. 'Elsa' interrupted, 'I do not like him. I can look at him now because his is not in my face; he is far from me!' Henk did not take this into consideration, and proceeded to choose a representative for Elsa's mother. The 'mother' was invited to face her 'daughter', but the 'daughter' did not show any interest in the 'mother'. Henk said to 'Elsa', 'You feel a strong connection to your mother.' 'Elsa' looked at the woman, then at Henk, and told him in a calm voice, 'I like her, but I'm not strongly connected.' The facilitator proceeded to move 'the children' to stand between 'Elsa' and 'Marcel', saying, 'You are a family', to which 'Elsa' responded, looking at Marcel, 'He is not my family!' Henk interpreted this to mean that now, when her mother was standing behind her, giving her more support, 'Elsa' did not see 'Marcel' as part of her family. He suggested that this is the case for many adopted men of colour who marry white Dutch women – there is continuous disrespect by their wives and in-laws. After this, the constellation was dismantled.

At the end of the day, while we were helping Henk and Marla to clean the room, the woman who had represented Elsa approached Henk and told him that he had misinterpreted what she was feeling during the session; that, in fact, she had had no sense of deep connection with her 'mother', and that she had felt afraid of her 'husband' and did not want to be near him. 'This is,' she continued, 'a bit funny, because outside of the constellation, I think Marcel is a very nice man.' Henk dismissed her comments, saying that it is best not to talk about what happened at the constellation and that she should go home, have a long shower and a massage if possible, and forget everything that happened on that day. Dissatisfied with his answer, she left the venue. Most of the participants complained about feeling exhausted and having tension in their muscles, and several participants agreed with one woman who said, 'I always feel so confused after these sessions, both in my mind and my body and still whole and complete.' While Henk had offered a suggestion to the woman who had represented 'Elsa' as to how to relax after the session, he did not offer similar suggestions to the others.

Following the session, Dragojlovic wrote to the participants, inviting them to share their experiences with her. Out of the 25 people who had attended, one woman wrote back to say that the experience had been devastating for her, and she was sure it had had the same effect on many others. However, the woman did not describe what she meant by 'devastating', and Dragojlovic never heard back from her. Out of the 14 people who had their questions constellated, eight wrote back to Dragojlovic months later, and all of them reported that their lives had changed considerably in the time since, but that they did not have a clear understanding of how such changes had occurred or whether they were related to the FCT session at all. Two people reported that they had felt a need to undergo intense counselling, which took several months to work on the 'trauma effects' of the session. In many ways, the responses of the participants were similar to how many of Dragojlovic's other interlocutors described the effects of the FCT sessions they undertaken.

In Dragojlovic's conversation with Henk following the session, Henk commented that FCT sessions that are focused on adoptees are very demanding both on the participants and on himself, as they often bring up his own adoption-related trauma. When Dragojlovic asked him about Elsa's representative's disagreement with his interpretation, he extended the argument he made at the session, adding that he knew Marcel and his situation well. Considering Henk's dismissal of Elsa's representative's feelings, Dragojlovic's asked, 'Does that mean that the knowing field is not always right, or that, perhaps, Marcel can be violent and Elsa was genuinely afraid of him?' Henk provided no answer. Dragojlovic's next question, about whether he had had a follow-up session with the participants, of whom many were obviously significantly distressed, he emphasised that it is not up to the facilitator to do that, and that what happened at the session must not be discussed afterwards in an attempt to enhance the session's effectiveness. Such an approach is intriguing, given that the driving force behind FCT is the revelation of hidden dynamics – yet what has been revealed must not be spoken about.

Bodily affectivity

What characterises the FCT session ethnographically described in this chapter, which is similar to many other FCT sessions Dragojlovic has attended, was an attitude that suffering and re-traumatisation will bring relief and the release of difficult emotions, and will clarify one's behaviour and free one from unwanted attachments to the past. In other words, re-traumatisation and intense suffering enacted through intersubjective and intercorporeal radical affectivity are not seen as regressive. In line with this, FCT sessions are expected to bring about self-transformation, reduce adoptees' sense of emotional distress and enhance a sense of self-sovereignty. As such, FCT workshops serve as an affective *economy of caring*, where the human body is understood in its capacity to affect and be affected, and intense emotional distress as states that create possibilities for self-transformation. While analyzing bodily affectivity and intersubjective healing, it is useful to recall the scholarly literature on affect. Affect has been described as autonomous, nonrepresentational, trans-subjective, immaterial or non-conscious (Blackman & Venn, 2010; Massumi, 2002; Seigworth & Gregg, 2010; Thrift, 2008), and refers to processes that circulate among bodies (Blackman, 2012; Brennan, 2004). Affect can also be understood as a 'state of being'; as an 'exchange' that has 'an energetic dimension' (Brennan 2004). Following Seigworth and Gregg's (2010) argument that bodies are not stable things or entities, Lisa Blackman (2012, p. 1) cogently argues that 'rather than talk about bodies, we might instead talk of brain-body-world entanglements.' Her conceptual proposition is crucially important when approaching the FCT method as a therapeutic modality that treats the lived body with intersubjective and intercorporeal capacities, rather than as a singular psychological subject. This also reminds us of what we seek to posit in this book and through all our case studies more broadly – that suffering lies across, not within, and that singularity is a normative construct, that limits and delimits the subject, and is a form of suffering in and of itself.

While, as we discussed in Chapter 4, non-FCT *For Adoptees* meetings are self-reflective attempts to engage with the affectivity of narratives, matters and things which form constitutive elements of the adoptees' negative feelings, FCT sessions are concerned with uncovering what is pre-reflective and pre-cognitive. Many of Dragojlovic's interlocutors (whether facilitators or clients at *For Adoptees*) agreed that the FCT sessions are a useful supplement to the conversations they have at *For Adoptees* meetings or other 'talking therapies' they undergo. For most of the FCT clients Dragojlovic spoke with, the body's affective, intersubjective and intercorporeal capacity ('to stand for someone else and feel the other's feelings'; 'to see another person acting and saying things you know but are not able to articulate') stood as a major point of transformation of the self, as well as of interpersonal relations and of their understanding of what it means to be human. Here, affect is re-worked through an FCT session, being at the same time intentional (accepting to suspend one's own will to stand as a representative) and nonintentional ('feeling like a loving father' for Nadia; 'being afraid of Marcel' for the representative of his wife; 'not wanting to look at the biological daughter' for Annelies' 'birth mother'). Affectivity here is also contested, as it is aligned with cultural and social expectations and presumptions (the lost father showing affection to the adopted daughter urgently needing his attention; Elsa's representative being frightened by a black man), but also in contrast to them (the 'birth mother' not showing any interest in her biological daughter, Annelies).

Similarly, the ways in which the participants interpreted their feelings describes the human body not as a static, bounded entity, but clearly with the capacity for intersubjective and intercorporeal interactions. The representative of Nadia's father, for example, reported to Dragojlovic afterwards that he felt affection for Nadia when he was representing her father, but felt afraid and uncomfortable after the session, when she still took him for her father. Similarly, Elsa's representative felt frightened while representing Marcel's wife, reporting to Dragojlovic later on that the fright she felt was a confirmation of the power of FCT to make you 'feel other people's feelings.' 'I was sort of sceptical about this whole thing', she told me, 'but feeling that urgency to run across the room towards the entrance from a person I had only met that morning, even though was a very nice person, changed something in me . . . Changed the way I see the world now. And you know, after the session, I also felt he was a nice man.' Here, we can clearly see what affect theorists have been arguing for some time; that 'we are not self-contained in terms of our energies', and that the transmission of affect occurs when 'energies of one person . . . enter directly into another' (Brennan, 2004, p. 6).

As we have seen, the ways in which affectivity is given meaning and qualified varies. In the ethnographic case study described in this chapter, this is particularly significant in the case of Marcel and the way that the facilitator interpreted (and potentially misinterpreted) bodily affectivity based on his experience and on his understanding of racialisation in Dutch society. As Henk argued, and as Drago-jlovic had heard from many of her other interlocutors, non-white male adoptees are often faced with the racialised images of the 'dangerous black man' or the 'meek Asian man'. In this case, however, such experiences serve as a disciplinary form of understanding the inequalities of racialization by not allowing for an interpretation in which a non-white male adoptee might be in some way threatening to his wife and children.

As Teresa Brennan (2004) argues, affects can enhance or deplete. We have seen that in the case of Annelies, where her 'birth mother's' refusal to acknowledge her produced a depleting affect, as it did in the case of Nadia, when the facilitator asked for a representative of her adopted father. Similarly, we have seen how Andreas' music and the lyrics of the songs he was performing had a depleting effect on most of the participants, enhancing their painful and distressful feelings (especially in Nadia and the other participants who left the session as a result). As Andreas' music was meant to attune the participants to their concerns and bring them closer to the emotional states from which they were perceived to be more capable to access the pre-reflective and pre-cognitive, we can see the value ascribed to enhancing the plethora of feelings associated with suffering. It is this affectivity of suffering, anguish and grief that those involved in the FCT session were aiming to re-work, affectively and intercorporeally.

While most of Dragojlovic's interlocutors valued the discussions, they shared at *For Adoptees* meetings and the more formal 'talking therapies' they had undergone, they also argued that these were not enough. Many of them mentioned having lurking feeling of deep-seated 'pain' and 'discomfort' which was beyond comprehension, or a feeling of 'not being in your body', 'being numb', 'not being able to feel', 'being paralysed', 'having a continuous sense of absence', and so on – as if an important part of themselves was inaccessible, and as if the mind and the body were disconnected. Due to such feelings, Dragojlovic's interlocutors reported that they needed to 'feel'; to 'experience' – in other words, they needed a somatic intervention in order to achieve their desired self-transformation. For Annelies and Nadia, the intensity of the pain they felt during the session was described as a 'cathartic release', as 'finally being able to breathe fully again'; as being able to 'feel whole'.

Conclusion

In this chapter, we have discussed the *For Adoptees* group method as an example of radical affective politics, and noted how this method aims to open up a space for the exploration of the creative possibilities inherent in questioning the normative demands posed on adoptees' subjecthood. We also noted how it problematises the normalisation of care relations as harmonious and devoid of power relations. The FCT session that we have discussed in this chapter operates under somewhat similar aims as the *For Adoptees* group method, and posits that the evocation of suffering and negative emotions can produce opportunities for creative transformation. In this way, the FCT session we ethnographically explored illuminates the body's capacity to affect and be affected, both intentionally and non-intentionally, as a simultaneous exchange and transmission that urges us to pay more attention to the relational aspects of subject formation. Moreover, the case study presented demonstrates how negative feelings can be approached as affective processes that can be re-worked intercorporeally; as processes that have the ability to lead towards desired self-transformation. Thus, the affective atmosphere of suffering, the intensity of the intersubjective exchanges and the sense of mutual healing were understood to have a reintegrating, focalising capacity, and a sense of bringing the 'fragmented self' into a state of 'wholeness'.

This case study urges us to think about suffering not in terms of the individual subject, but rather, as comprising assemblages of bodies, technologies (in this case of healing), discourses, practices and performances. Our intention is not to argue either for or against the healing modality presented here, but instead to note these practices of healing unavoidably draw our attention to the value ascribed to negative affect and their evocation. Here, suffering as negative affect is both the solution to and a site for suffering. This suggests that suffering is and can be a process of becoming.

Notes

1 The names of all interlocutors, as well as the sites and locations where the session occurred, have been altered in order to protect the anonymity of Dragojlovic's interlocutors.
2 The concept of self-sovereignty has been used in feminist struggles over women's bodily rights. For a detailed discussion of these struggles, see Steinberg (1997).

3 Some practitioners argue that such intergenerational influence spans between three to seven generations, depending on the individual case.
4 Pseudonym.

References

Ahmed, S. (2010). *The Promise of Happiness*. Durham, NC: Duke University Press.

Blackman, L. (2008). *The Body: The Key Concepts*. Oxford, New York: Berg.

Blackman, L. (2012). *Immaterial Bodies: Affect, Embodiment, Mediation*. Thousand Oaks, CA: Sage.

Blackman, L. (2015). Affective politics, debility and hearing voices: Towards a feminist politics of ordinary suffering. *Feminist Review*, 111(4) pp. 25–41.

Blackman, L. & Venn, C. (2010). Affect. *Body & Society*, 16(1), pp. 1–6.

Böszörményi-Nagy, I. & Spark, G. (1973). *Invisible Loyalties: Reciprocity in Intergenerational Family Therapy*. Hagerstown: Harper & Row.

Brennan, T. (2004). *The Transmission of Affect*. Ithaca and London: Cornell University Press.

Cant, S. & Sharma, U. (1999). *A New Medical Pluralism: Complementary Medicine, Doctors, Patients and the State*. London, New York: Routledge.

Cohen, D. B. (2006). 'Family Constellations': An innovative systemic phenomenological group process from Germany. *The Family Journal: Counselling and Therapy for Couples and Families*, 14(3), pp. 226–233.

Csordas, J. T. (2008). Intersubjectivity and intercorporeality. *Subjectivity*, 22, pp. 110–121.

Cvetkovich, A. (2012). *Depression: A Public Feeling*. Durham, NC: Duke University Press.

Davies, J. (2012). *The Importance of Suffering: The Value and Meaning of Emotional Discontent*. London, New York: Routledge.

Dragojlovic, A. (2014). The search for sensuous geographies of absence: Indisch mediation of loss. *Bijdragen tot de Taal-, Land- en Volkenkunde* (*Journal of the Humanities and Social Sciences of Southeast Asia*), 170(4), pp. 473–503.

Dragojlovic, A. (2015). Affective geographies: Intergenerational hauntings, bodily affectivity and multiracial subjectivities. *Subjectivity*, 8, pp. 315–334.

Dragojlovic, A. (2016). *Beyond Bali: Subaltern Citizens and Post-Colonial Intimacy*. Amsterdam: Amsterdam University Press.

Ernst, W. (2014). *Plural Medicine, Tradition and Modernity*. London, New York: Routledge.

Halberstam, J. J. (2011). *The Queer Art of Failure*. Durham, NC: Duke University Press.

Heller, T., Lee-Treweek, G., Katz, J., Stone, J. & Spurr, S., eds. (2005). *Perspectives on Complementary and Alternative Medicine: A Reader*. London, New York: Routledge.

Hellinger, B., Weber, G. & Beaumont, H. (1998). *Love's Hidden Symmetry: What Makes Love Work in Relationships*. Phoenix: Zeig, Tucker and Theisen.

Keegan, L. (2000). *Healing with Complementary & Alternative Therapies*. London: Delmar Cengage Learning.

Keleman, S. (1981). *Your Body Speaks its Mind*. Berkeley, CA: Center Press.

Keleman, S. (1985). *Emotional Anathomy: The Structure of Experience*. Berkley, CA: Center Press.

Latour, B. (2004). How to talk about about the body? The normative dimensions of science studies. *Body & Society*, 10(2–3), pp. 205–230.

Love, H. (2007). *Feeling Backward: Loss and the Politics of Queer History*. Cambridge: Harvard University Press.

Massumi, B. (2002). *Parables for the Virtual: Movement, Affect, Sensation*. Durham, NC: Duke University Press.

Mol, A. (2002). *The Body Multiple: Ontology in Medical Practice*. Durham, NC: Duke University Press.

Moreno, J. L. (1945). *Psychodrama*. New York: Beacon.

Ruggie, M. (2004). *Marginal to Mainstream: Alternative Medicine in America*. Cambridge: Cambridge University Press.

Seigworth, G. J. & Gregg, M. (2010). An inventory of shimmers. In Gregg, M. &

Seigworth, G. J., eds, *The Affect Theory Reader*. Durham, NC: Duke University Press, pp. 1–27.

Sheldrake, R. (1995). *The Presence of the Past: Morphic Resonance and the Habits of Nature*. Rochester, VT: Park Street Press.

Stacey, J. (2000). The global within. In Franklin, S., Lury, C. & Stacey, J., eds, *Global Nature, Global Culture*. London: Sage, pp. 97–145.

Steinberg, D. (1997). *Bodies in Glass: Genetics, Eugenics, Embryo Ethics*. Manchester: Manchester University Press.

Sutherland, J.-A., Polman, M. M. & Pendelton, B. F. (2003). Religion, spirituality and alternative health practices: The baby boomer and Cold War cohorts. *Journal of Religion and Health*, 42(4), pp. 315–338.

Thrift, N. (2008). *Non-Representational Theory: Space, Politics, Affect*. New York: Routledge.

Wekker, G. (2016). *White Innocence: Paradoxes of Colonialism and Race*. Durham, NC: Duke University Press.

Wilard, B. E. (2005). Feminist interventions in biomedical discourse: An analysis of the rhetoric of integrative medicine. *Women's Studies in Communication*, 28(1), pp. 115–148.

6   Suffering survivorship

Dilemmas of survival,
wilful subjects and the
moral economy of dying

Introduction

Daniel: Yeah, I survive, oh yeah. I'm not going to let the bastard get me for
nothing. I would think it's got a lot to do with; a lot of people just don't
realise no matter how far you go, you've still got a choice. [Advanced
cancer, Australia]

In this chapter, we seek to explore some less documented, and perhaps more
unsettling, aspects of cancer survivorship. This exploration is set within a context of 'survivorship' more broadly as a dominant discursive field, a powerful
cultural device, and a technique of capture; it is at once a biophysical reality, a
cultural practice, a social role, a perceived human quality and a normative facet
of our social milieu. Survivorship is ubiquitous in the cancer field, espoused by
a wide array of organisations, research institutions, practitioner governing bodies, pharmaceutical and political interests.[1] Survivorship emerges from our social
fabric, articulating our modern sense of mastery over affliction, medical successes
in delaying death and slowing ageing, and our dread of our inevitable demise.
Survivorship practice produces, and is produced by, relations of wilfulness, hope,
dread, obligation, reciprocity and somatic necessity. It is a historical, economic
and political act and imperative, emergent from relations of citizens to the modern
State, to their family and to their responsibilities. It is part – the finale, perhaps –
of the neoliberal social contract to be a productive member of society; to survive
is to be uniquely human in the cultural imaginary. To capitulate to 'the bastard',
as Daniel puts it above, is to yield to the pressure of affliction and somatic decay.
Such acts are the antithesis of the practice of survivorship, and indeed, the articulation of a 'good life' (Berlant, 2011; Steinberg, 2015). To not be allowed to yield,
to concede, to 'lose the battle', however, offers up new and important forms of
suffering.

One of the questions that guide our analysis in this chapter – and one of the
core struggles our participants have experienced in seeking to live with their
cancer – is how the survivorship agenda resonates with the inevitability human
mortality. What happens at the inevitable clash of ambition and insatiable desire

for perseverance (from us and/or others) and the inevitability of our demise? Survivorship is part of the cultural ammunition against an end-point, against surrender. It articulates the cultural assumption that death is a 'necessary evil' in a mortal world – unavoidable, inevitable but ultimately unthinkable. While this pre-text to our analysis below may be viewed as being *unfair on* proponents of survivorship – and even survivors themselves, whoever these may be – this is not our intention. Rather, we seek to understand the modern survivorship imperative and its often-concealed pernicious impacts. From a cultural desire for longevity emerges simplistic ideas around survival – what it means, achieves and offers to the person (and those around them). What is required to counter such simplicities, we posit, is a more nuanced perspective on survivorship, one that reveals its many faces, and one that 'outs' survivorship as existing at the intersection of the discursive, relational, somatic and affective. This perspective should identify how feelings like hope are more than personal experiences or expressions of an internal life world, which has surfaced. Rather, as Ahmed (2014) observes, in other arenas, survivorship settles on people, often in incomplete or uncomfortable ways, producing or encouraging, as it were, particular forms of affect in the context of different forms of affliction (Sointu, 2015). The purpose or aim of this approach is not to suggest that a person's feelings and forms of knowing around survival are somehow illegitimate. Rather, we argue that such feelings are at the nexus of the discursive, the normative and social (Ahmed, 2004a); this understanding neither separates, nor diminishes the significance of, the emotive in cancer contexts. The problem emerges within the field of survivorship when such things (individual feelings, expressions, desires) are seen as independent from the social milieu or when such connectivities are concealed, reifying the character of the individual and concealing the contribution of the social field. For example, it is assumed someone *has* the will to survive; or, that someone has *lost* the will to live. Such statements – captured in the erstwhile maxim 'where there's a will, there's a way' – conceal survivorship as sociality, as a *practice* produced concurrently by institutions, practitioners, families, partners, children as well as afflicted subjects (Illouz, 2007). Survivorship is a site of resistance, horror, disdain and dread, as well as many other 'productive' feelings for many who are facing terminal illnesses and even death.

In the context of cancer, which we focus on here, survivorship is the overarching discursive field that subjects must/will navigate. As people edge toward death, they must somehow forge a path through a complex terrain – the narrative of resilience, coping, persisting, healing – the cultural norms of survivorship (Stacey, 1997). The affective dimensions experienced and forms of suffering therein can be profound (as we shall show here) and offer considerable insight into the complicity of survivorship in suffering but also enmeshment in meaning-making and character-building at the end of life. This 'dark side' – the Janus-faced feature of cancer survivorship – is embedded in a broader context of the new subjects of neoliberal sociality or what Steinberg (2015) calls 'the "neoliberal body-reflexive" ethic that infuses the representational field of cancer' (p. 20) offering a duplicity in its promises to the subject with cancer. Whilst we acknowledge that survivorship as a cultural discourse operated well before the emergence of neoliberalism, it remains the case that it has additional purchase within this socio-cultural, economic and political context, as articulated in Steinberg's (2015) of the cancer patient:

> The social conditions of her life, even the biological conditions of her life, are not consequential, or not as consequential, as her personal determination and will. Her life models ours. And ours, as a logical corollary, are obliged to model hers. This is the quintessential neoliberal subject . . . body-affective imperatives that are ruthlessly estranging and in which self-assertion is phantasmatically secured through its obverse – subjection, transferred agency, denial, distantiation . . . it is powerfully evident that the cancer patient is no longer a metaphor of hopelessness, or corruption, or tragedy or shame.
>
> (p. 21)

As intonated in Steinberg's depiction, whilst survivorship is all too often positioned as an admirable human trait, human characteristic and individual act, it is in fact a much more (potentially) malevolent force that is inter-subjectively instituted rather than individually chosen. In this chapter, we will offer a reading of cancer survivorship as composed of mixed qualities; as being potential and concurrently enabling and disabling, personally inscribing and collectively mediated; but also as producing erroneous distinctions between self, disease, the body and the social. Cancer survivorship is often mistaken for *the potential* of a subject – the capacity to choose, to be autonomous, to be responsible, to persevere. Yet, it is often the normative quality of requests by others for subjects to *be* this way. Technologies, expertise and ideologies emerge from different sectors of society (e.g. medicine, alternative therapies, self-help, psychotherapy) to facilitate the ambitions and desires of survivorship (see also Illouz, 2008).

Furthermore, there is indeed no doubt that many techniques are of enduring value and comfort to those who are living with cancer. As we will also show in this chapter, though, some such practices emerging from, and surrounding, survivorship discourse valorise the qualities of the person, the act, and in doing so misattribute capacities (usually, to either mind, body or self). Such practices may involve willing disease away, self-healing, transcending affliction, repairing the body and self, to improve and get better – and to *do better*. These qualities of the human subject are often taken 'out of context' in line with the problematic cultural individualisation of illness and affliction. In her book *Cruel Optimism* (2011), Lauren Berlant engages in the broader cultural practices which inform such social scripts, but which are helpful for understanding certain facets of the normative qualities and cultural underpinnings of survivorship. This includes the emergent optimistic imperative – a sense that being dutiful will indeed result in what one deserves. For Berlant, there is a cruelty within such relations when

> the object/scene that ignites a sense of possibility actually makes it impossible to attain the expansive transformation for which a person or a people risks

striving; and doubly, it is cruel insofar as the very pleasures of being inside a relation have become sustaining regardless of the content of the relation, such that a person or a world finds itself bound to a situation of profound threat that is, at the same time, profoundly confirming.

(2011, p. 2)

Berlant's observation provides a useful platform for embarking on an analysis of the potential entrapment of survivorship, and the potentially problematic outcomes of therapeutic strategies perpetuated within survivorship discourse. The logics of survivorship may at one time be incredibly sustaining, and profoundly confirming for people with cancer and those around them, yet they may jar with others forms of knowing, or at worst, be impossible to obtain. Often inadvertently, healthcare practitioners, in seeking to grapple with their own and their patients' emotions regarding cancer and death (i.e. fear, disappointment, hopelessness, loss of control, shame and progressive decay), utilise survivorship in such ways to turn these emotions of affliction 'on their head' (i.e. to inspire hope, agency, self-autonomy). But, we posit here, to what end and for whose desires? There are considerable questions surrounding whether the ambitions of survivorship and its respective institutions, technologies, practices and norms ameliorate suffering, and indeed, offer a relation of cruelty. Or perhaps, it does both, and requires reconsideration to capture the complexities of the juggernaut of survivorship. We need to question whether the survivorship 'industry' (industries of hope, self-healing, self-care, self-actualisation) entails a selective utilisation of culturally valued expressions and performances. Certainly such ideologies offer an intriguing contrast to the forms of biophysical reductionism that many cancer patients have been subject to for years before they are deemed terminal, or indeed, to be dying. Yet, while perhaps the rise of self-healing and self-care may be light relief in the context of disease-centricity – to no longer be at the 'will of their bodies', as Frank (2002) articulates it, the construction of self-as-agent (of one's survival or demise), may offer a new form of reductionism, inadvertently reinforcing cultural models of individuation and the qualities therein (Illouz, 2008).

The purpose of this chapter is to present survivorship – of and with advanced cancer – as an assemblage of medical, alternative and cultural knowledge and practices; bodies, technologies and the somatic; and, emotions and feelings (cf. Blackman, 2008), recognising that these factors are necessarily intertwined. We argue that the affective dimensions of survivorship – including hope, wilfulness, fear, dread, optimism and shame – emerge from such assemblages; or what (Blackman, 2008) might call the 'brain-body-world nexus'. That the personal – the seemingly 'individual feelings' – articulate the broader cultural interpretations attached to people bodies and places (Sointu, 2015). We view survivorship practice as articulating ideas about value (capital); and that feelings and somatic experiences are entangled with (to a greater or lesser degree) such scripts, emerging as an estrangement or affiliation (which shifts over time as affliction evolves). Yet we also view feelings as unwieldy, and indeed unsettling, as they/we resist the 'things' that attempt to settle on us (e.g. 'death is coming', 'acceptance is transcendent', 'stoic survival is reflective of character').

While the emotions of survival (or dying, as it were) are often 'treated' as personal and individual, they are not. They are, in fact, circulating beliefs, experiences, desires and feelings of individuals and collectives. They are the partial articulation of collective feelings of the cultural attachment to life and longevity (and dread that such things are no longer possible). It is *not* that the individual does not matter, and that what the individual does *cannot matter*; but that the survivorship agenda and its affective dimensions are the outcome of cultural discourse, professional desire, the somatic, technological possibilities, and embodied ways of knowing (Blackman & Venn, 2010). The survivorship agenda involves tussles between the limits and possibilities of these spheres; that different forms of wilfulness – from professionals, families and patients – exert pressure in certain directions, allow certain subject positions to prosper, and require certain forms of expression and indeed repression. In outlining the complexities of cancer survivorship we seek to emphasise the *estranged subjects* of the survivorship space (Steinberg, 2015). What we mean by this is the practice, articulation and ways of knowing and doing that unsettle established modes of living and dying. Much of these understandings are based on disconnection between person, the social, or body and the cultural, and the outcome of the reification of splits that disconnect spheres that illustrate the very tensions and complexities that cancer patients face in experiencing affliction and embarking on survivorship (whether to survive or surviving until death). Steinberg (2015) touches on such things in her discussion of 'the bad patient, she who might not be interested in marching forward (or be able to do so), who might not be invested in life at any cost, or perhaps even at all, she who is "not brave" . . .' (p. 21). What Steinberg usefully points to is the dynamic of estrangement in the midst of the discursive production of the cancer patient, but also the strength of will exerted by Others in and around cancer patients, to keep 'marching forward' (see also Ahmed, 2014). What occurs, we posit below, is a series of tussles around ways of *knowing* (intuitive, embodied, lay, expert) and *being* (surviving, dying, resilience, hopelessness) as a cancer patient and as the subject of care, producing, as it were, complex affective dimensions.

Notes on fieldwork

This chapter draws on several studies led by Broom in 2004–2005 (UK, diary-based), 2006–2007 (Australia, interview-based), 2011–2014 (Australia, interview-based) and 2015–present (Australia, interview-based). These studies involved cancer patients with advanced or end-stage disease, who were either receiving treatment for metastatic or incurable disease, or palliative care (in-patient or out-patient).[2] We draw across these data sets for two purposes. The first is for methodological reasons. The studies offer a mix of individual interviews and diary case studies, filled out by the participants over a one month period, and this provides both snapshot and temporal insights into survivorship and the dynamics of suffering. The second is that each of these studies raised consistent and persistent themes around survivorship. While the 2004–2005 and 2006–2007 studies were focused on engagement with complementary medicines by cancer patients, the 2011–2014 and 2015–present studies focused on the broader, lived experience of advanced cancer care. Despite being distributed over the course of more than a decade, each of these raised connected ideas about personal and interpersonal struggles around survivorship, moral tensions around what *should* and *could* be achieved by 'cancer patients' and forms of suffering therein. The diaries provided an interesting departure from the interview material, offering a temporal inflection, and removing to some extent the (direct) presence of the researcher in the narrative. The interviews were completed either in the participant's homes or in a private area within a clinical environment. The diaries were completed over a one-month period so as to not overly burden the participants already faced with a likely terminal diagnosis of cancer.

Facing mortality, making survivorship

The participants' dilemmas around survivorship often first emerged in their interactions with their oncologist or treating doctor. A critical moment tended to be the clinical disclosure of their 'terminal' status. This moment offered powerful clinical discourse, usually around futility, inevitability, death as determined and inevitable. This moment had complex ripple effects across the lives and futures of the participants. This particular moment of discussion articulated the contrast between cultural desire, clinical knowing and affective, embodied lay desire, and ambitions for the future. As evident below, the interviews were filled with mixed feelings about being exposed to clinical predictions and the spectre of death; with a consistent questioning of clinical discourse, and resistance to the idea of terminality and futility. Claims of 'being in denial', being 'a difficult patient' and so forth, were regularly recounted as their doctors' views on their practices of resistance in clinical encounters, reflecting an affect of estrangement; an undermining interpersonal dynamic whereby desire is prominent (desire of patient for a *different trajectory*; desire of doctor for a capacity to *be potent*). Specifically, the somatic situation and clinical knowledge therein emerges as mutually exclusive of the desire of both parties:

Belinda: I think knowing what the doctors have said prognosis-wise, and I know they're probably right, but I don't want them to be right. That's why I said, I'm making a five-year plan. I think you have to do that. I've seen so many people say, 'The doctors have said I should be dead by now.' Then they're at home expecting to die any minute, and they don't . . . You can't stop living because somebody's told you, 'You're going to die' . . . If I can't keep doing what I'm able to do then is that going to make me die sooner? . . . The doctors aren't always right. [Female, cancer, 2015–present study, Australia]

Ricky: [. . .] For the doctors to turn up at the ward at the [hospital] and say, 'Ricky, this is the results of all your tests, you have cancer, it's terminal, we can't do anything for you. We recommend that you go home now and prepare yourself for the end, because it's nigh.' Which is basically the words he [oncologist] said . . . I'll never forget that. He and a team of six other doctors sat there in front of my wife and I and just told us to go home and get ready to die. That was straight out pretty brutal . . . And he got up and he shook my hand and he said, 'I haven't got any better news for you, see you later,' and him and his team of doctors walked out of the room. Now I don't know whether you can imagine what that might be like, it's dreadful. So my wife and I, we sat there and we looked at each other and we both burst into tears and all that sort of stuff. [Male, advanced cancer, 2011–2014 study, Australia]

Joan: [. . .] when I've spoken to both my GP and the oncologist at the [hospital], I talk about remission, 'what's the chances of my remission?' . . . my own GP was [like] 'you're in denial,' and I said, 'I'm not in denial.' I know I've got cancer but I'm [not] going to die from cancer . . . [Female, advanced cancer, 2011–2014 study, Australia]

Eileen: [. . .] the first thing he ever said to me when I sat down was, 'I'm not going cure you,' and that, I think, was very deflating to me. Like I knew it wasn't going to go away in my bones, but no one really wants it said to you that bluntly the first time you meet him kind of thing. And that was the last time I saw him for six months because he wasn't there, he was on holidays, he was on conference and things like that . . . I think what he wanted was someone he could cure, so I kind of wasn't his main target area, so felt like shoved to the background. [Female, advanced cancer, 2011–2014 study, Australia]

We turn to wilfulness in greater detail below, but the exchanges between doctor and 'patient' at the point of an initial prognosis of terminal disease, are often the platforms for competing forms of will (i.e. clinical, expert, patient, lay, survivor) which necessarily produce a range of affective responses for different subjects in the clinical encounter. Like the rod in Ahmed's (2014, pp. 136–137) examination of the Brothers Grimm's fairy tale *A Wilful Child*, clinical knowledge, techniques and motions – including prognostic knowledge, clinical predictions, medical discourses of possibility–pacify subjects but *also* render the persons/patients wilful. Being told they will die often 'kick-started' the will to live. The therapeutic encounter was thus regularly described as a tussle over forms of will (clinical/lay), and often prompted survivorship trajectories. We note that it is not that prognostic information cannot be useful, important or even vital for people with cancer and those surrounding them. Rather, we seek to problematise prognostic encounters as merely the exchange of information about the subject's disease; rather, that such encounters are an amalgamation of discourse, desire and emotions (*as well as* epidemiological data – the so-called 'bell curve' of survival). While above we present a series of excerpts on the tussles between doctors and patients over the futility of further treatment, the reverse dynamic was also prevalent in other narratives. That is, the valorisation of the need for 'fight', 'persistence' and the value of overcoming affliction from the perspective of health professionals. The participants would often report being told by their oncologists that 'it's up to you now', 'those who are positive live longer', or 'maintaining positivity is what you should do'. These rhetorical strategies and ideological positions reflect two sides of the 'cancer survivorship coin' with important consequences for its subjects and their families. They also are a manifestation of the contradictory demands circulating our cultural milieu (e.g. to accept/to survive; to cope/to let go; to fight/ to release; to acknowledge/to forge on). They are in turn key influences on the lived experience of cancer and the end of life. Following Ahmed (2004a), we posit that these and the many other accounts of the therapeutic encounter further illustrate the fact that emotions around survivorship are *not* private matters, or that they come from within and then move outward toward others. Rather, we posit that emotions – in this case, around the 'proper' response to cancer – 'create the very effect of the surfaces or boundaries of bodies and worlds' (Ahmed, 2004a, p. 117). Without discrediting counter-narratives, we could ask what can be said or achieved by expressions like 'it's not my time', 'I will do what I feel despite what they say', and I will not 'let the bastard get me'.

Similarly, it is unclear what statements such as 'positive people do well' or 'it's up to you now' may also achieve within therapeutic encounters. In dialogue with these participants, it was clear that very often survivorship rhetoric and practice was underpinned by deep sense of fear – a dominant form of affect and aspect of internal suffering for those facing a terminal prognosis and the end of their lives. This does not remove or disallow the credibility of such statements, but offers a more nuanced take on what lies beneath. There are many questions here, but some are: what produces fear in this context? What purpose does it serve? And, from where does it arise in our cultural and social histories?

Fear and survivorship

It would come as little surprise that the narratives gathered in the studies provide a wide-ranging series of reflections on fear. While not all participants in the studies discussed fear of death and dying, or indeed suffering at the end of life, most did, and thus fear was a prevalent affective dimension driving their accounts of, and acts of, survivorship (whether aimed at cure, securing longevity, or just 'lasting another day or week'). This is not to say that they were deluded or in denial. Rather, their practices of survivorship are informed by cultural ideas and social practices, many of which imbue a fear of mortality and death. Fear, in the interviews, was regularly articulated in relation to a wide range of factors, with some verbatim examples being: 'is there hell or nothing?', 'will I suffer at the end?', 'will I become dependent on others in my final days?', 'I can't give up', 'will it be messy?'. Their narratives of fear articulated the nexus of survival and cultural discourse around personal character (resilience) and the meaning of death (redemption, judgement day, sin) and biophysical realities and landscapes of cancer on the body. Below are just some examples of the assemblage/assembling of fear, often drawing from broader cultural understandings of the meaning of death.

Fears formed and inform people's survivorship trajectories. Such accounts are another reminder that survivorship (and its affective dimension) does not occur just because of an innate human need to prevail; rather, it arises out of cultural, social, historical, economic and political imperatives which are transformed into forms of affect in people's lives. Fear produces dilemmas around resisting death, not giving up, and the need to prevail over affliction, regardless of 'the odds':

Eileen: . . . I think sometimes if you want to give up you just look at how far you've actually come. But I'm super-scared of dying . . . I was brought up a Catholic, I'm actually thinking about going to see a priest and ask, because I was brought up a Catholic so you've got that belief in hell. And I think of all the things I've done wrong, he's [God] not going to take me up to heaven. So that scares you a little bit, and then what scares me more is that there isn't anything and then all of this was just a big joke, this doesn't mean anything at all, like anything we've done, in the end it doesn't mean anything, so that's really scary too. [. . .] And you have to die terribly to get it [heaven] . . . [Female, advanced cancer, 2011–2014 study, Australia]

Barry: Well he [oncologist] wanted me to prepare for palliative care. And I said, 'have you got me ready for the box? Am I going to die next week?' And he said, 'no, we just want to prepare you for the future'.

Interviewer: How did you feel about that?

Barry: Well, I don't feel like death, I don't want death. [Male, advanced cancer, 2011–2014 study, Australia]

Diana: . . . it [advanced cancer] is very, very difficult because it's like a death sentence, of course. And I'm wondering when this is going to happen, it's been a big, big battle, it still is . . . you know you're going to die of it eventually, and you're wondering what is going to happen to you before. Death, I don't mind, but the suffering and all that, but they reassured me that they're going to drug me and all this sort of stuff. [Female, advanced cancer, 2011–2014 study, Australia]

As shown above, and in many of the other interviewees' accounts, fear was a stigmatised but palpable feeling. There was a certain degree of shame in fear (Probyn, 2004), whether embedded in perceived religious wrongdoings or ambiguities over salvation, or indeed, the awareness that one should be brave. But what is fear here? It is not simply a fear of an end. Rather, it is a product of cultural, historical and ideological logics which 'stick' to the subject, and which then become concealed in the logic of fear as a normal facet of facing our future (or lack thereof). As Ahmed (2004b) argues:

fear does not reside in a particular object or sign, and it is this lack of residence that allows [it to] slide across signs, and between bodies. This sliding becomes stuck only temporarily, in the very attachment of a sign to a body, whereby a sign sticks to a body by constituting it as the object of fear, a constitution taken on by the body, encircling it with a fear that *becomes its own.*

(p. 127; emphasis added)

While Ahmed is describing a very different dynamic, a malignancy acts in a similar fashion; fear does not reside in it, but it is constituted as the object of fear. In the narratives provided by interviewees, fear was deeply enmeshed in the expectation to 'die well', articulated by one participant as follows: 'my greatest fear is dying struggling, fighting. I don't want to fight, I mean, if the time comes.' This anticipatory anxiety took the form of a restlessness, which we posit, is an articulation of a complex assemblage.

Restlessness and wondering

Each period of data collection revealed interesting intersections of embodied experience, cultural discourse, medical knowledge and affect. One of the most revealing and consistently arising experiences was that of *restlessness*. Restlessness has been thoroughly 'explained' in the medical literature; and has been constructed as a normal facet of the dying process (e.g. Burke et al., 1991; White et al., 2007). As 'the body', it is said, prepares for death, then the 'normal' rhythms are unsettled as part of the preparation for one's imminent demise. For the participants in these studies, restlessness was much more than their 'bodies' preparing for death (as if such a somatic process could occur separately and automatically). Rather, it articulated their brain-body-world tussles. Restlessness challenged separations, incorporating a moving assemblage of cultural discourse (the push to survive, the push to accept), affliction (physical pain and discomfort), feelings (including hope, melancholia), and existential musings (desire for redemption, absolution). These moved in and out of one another, circulating around the collective (family, social group, clinical actors), being *produced by* the individual and the collective. A focus on the significance of restlessness may be usefully connected to Blackman's (2008) encouragement of us to consider how we 'think through the body' – and to in turn break down the physical, biological and social elements of the body. This, we posit, is pertinent to the interviews. As the interviewees' recount below, with death coming closer and 'survivorship' becoming increasingly difficult, he felt an acute form of constant restlessness:

Patrick: . . . to look at me you wouldn't think I'm going to cark it in the next three months, but yeah, just feeling a little down.

Interviewer: That must be really difficult.

Patrick: It's a horrible thought, to think you haven't got that long to go.

Interviewer: Can I ask how it's affecting things?

Patrick: Made me depressed, well, depression has set in. I feel very restless, not eating at the moment, you feel as though you want to sleep all the time, [and you] feel as though you can't [sleep]. Whereas I used to like being entertained before, used to like having company, now it's . . . gone the other way totally. It's more depressing than ever. [Male, advanced cancer, 2011–2014 study, Australia]

Angus: But I mean you know I've done it, I've *been* happy, I've got nothing else to do but survive until I die. [Male, advanced cancer, 2011–2014 study, Australia; *emphasis added*]

Kathryn: I think people get scared, [it comes] back to the, you get sick and you die, or you get sick and it goes away, and people don't like this hanging on . . . friends tend to dribble away as it goes, 'oh, she's still sick', you know and they don't get the *in between*. [Female, advanced cancer, 2011–2014 study, Australia; *emphasis added*]

Restlessness, here, articulates a range of factors relating to survivorship, and indeed, dying. Restlessness forms an important lay narrative; it moves across brain-body-world distinctions, circulating around the collective (see Chapter 1 for a discussion of the affective dilemmas of doctors and nurses) and rests on the person. Rather than merely being an automatic, physical processes – and one to be medicalised by sedation, benzodiazepine,[3] and so forth – it articulates cultural taboos, social obligations, individual desire and discontents as well as somatic trajectories (see also Blackman & Venn, 2010). Restlessness is thus a useful descriptor (when taken beyond its medical usage) as it does not pacify the body, disease, person, or collective and preclude the recognition of its assemblage. Rather, it reveals how experiences of individual (so-called 'normal') dying *becomes* rather than *is*.

Further, restlessness suggests that the culmination of discourse, moralities and expectations around surviving and dying. Restlessness, as articulated by these participants, is not merely a 'fact of dying'. This also resonates with what Blackman (2008) describes as 'a feeling body that presents a challenge to the kind of Cartesian dualism that produces the body as mere physical substance' (p. 4). It is worth considering the extent to which this relates to Blackman's (2008) notion of 'communicating bodies' and of the lived body (i.e. consideration of the body as experience, in terms of sensations and its relation to its 'outside'). An important facet of restlessness was not the underlying wondering of the participants about when their 'time was up' but fears around how this would be received by others around them (Probyn, 2004). Restlessness, in this context, articulates the dialectic of internal wonderings and external obligations, and illustrates how suffering in survivorship can operate:

Connie: Well if, I think that myself at times and then when I express it the others get very annoyed with me. So you know, you wonder at times whether the discomfort you have is worth it, but then you wonder well how much more life you're going to have and what kind of life you're going to live and whether it's going to be worthwhile. Yeah it's a very difficult decision to say 'no, I won't have the treatment.' [Female, advanced cancer, 2011–2014 study, Australia]

Erica: Oh, what a chore, living. I'd just as soon die.

Interviewer:	Really?
Erica:	Yep, I'd just as soon die. Yeah, I'm 85 and there's nothing more. There's nothing really in this life to sort of get excited about.
Interviewer:	Yeah?
Erica:	But anyhow I don't know, it doesn't look as though I am going to die.
Interviewer:	Right. Carrying on despite your best wishes.
Erica:	Whether I like it or not.
Interviewer:	Yeah? What do you think your husband and daughters would say?
Erica:	Oh they don't like that at all.
Interviewer:	Do you tell them that that's how you feel?
Erica:	Yeah, I tell them I feel like dying and they go, 'no, you can't do that!' And the grandchildren say, 'no, you can't do that!' [Female, advanced cancer, 2011–2014 study, Australia]

We continue later in this chapter to explore the dynamic of surviving in relation, but it is certainly worth reinforcing at this point that restlessness and surviving as a relation are closely connected. Restlessness is a useful explanatory mechanism for the inherent contradictions of survivorship. Despite the wonderings of the participants, often almost whispered in the interviews, restlessness articulated a sense of failure of will, a key dynamic which we explore below.

Wilfulness and resistance

What does it mean to be wilful in the context of living with cancer? Where does wilfulness come from? Should one will oneself through pain, suffering and progressive bodily decay; or to health and wellness? Wilfulness, we posit here, is much more than an emotive disposition, that is, a feeling. Rather, it is a social norm, cultural practice and relational activity. Such practices: 'mediate the relationship between the psychic and the social, and between the individual and the collective' (Ahmed, 2004a, p. 27). In the context of this chapter, the demands on individuals with cancer (to accept/survive; be stoic/peaceful; to resist) put *will* at centre stage in the survivorship field. In her book *Willful Subjects* (2014), Ahmed argues that 'if authority assumes the right to turn a wish into a command, then wilfulness is a diagnosis of the failure to comply with those whose authority is given' (p. 1). A question here is thus where authority lies in the cancer field – in the hands of the diagnosing doctors who say it is or is not futile; with those who espouse resilience and hope, whether doctors or other health professionals? Or does authority emerge from the broader the cultural valorisation of resilience, endurance and transcendence? Is it the *will* to live, to strive, to live on? Or perhaps authority is the will to die, and of one's own volition? In living with cancer, people move back and forth from and within such demands. Wilfulness is thus a complex assemblage of each and all of these demands.

What is interesting is how, again drawing on Ahmed (2004a), emotions are part of the production of coherence within the survivorship imperative. The fear of death and mortality – and the desire to illustrate strength of will – does not lie within the person, for example, it circulates our social milieu; it is a collective product (Probyn, 2004). Forms of authority have been established around these collective ideas and feelings – of the need for resilience and survival, confounded by the reasonableness of death and dying (it is, ultimately, a futile fight). The person – the subject – is thus faced with a confusing mix of collective feelings and contradictory requests to exert will. The narratives of these participants illustrate that these signs, scripts and normative structures do not necessarily sit well; they are awkwardly imposed on their (individual) desires, experiences and embodied forms of knowing. Below, we explore particular forms of wilfulness, and in later sections of this chapter, the estranged and often concealed forms of will that can emerge in cancer journeys:

Richard: . . . once you give up and well then there isn't any treatment that's going to fill in that gap anymore. And the reality is I haven't given up.

Interviewer: That's a very strong thing for you to . . .

Richard: Absolutely every day, part of my mantra: 'I will survive to celebrate my seventieth birthday.' I intend to see all three of my children happily married, I will hold all three of my grandchildren in my arms. It hasn't happened yet, it's a reality that I hold onto. You know, and once those have been achieved, well, I'll find something else. [Male, Advanced Cancer, 2011–2014 study, Australia]

Barry: Well I want to go on for as long as I can enjoying life and not sort of saying, 'well I've got cancer, I'm going to die.' And that is inevitable, but I don't want to lie down and accept it. I want to fight it, if you like, and be positive about it for as long as I can. But I don't know what's around the corner. [Male, advanced cancer, 2011–2014 study, Australia]

Susan: Yeah, and I know when I got into this business of being a cancer patient, truly, I felt like I was dying and I got sicker and sicker and sicker. I could have just have resigned myself at some mental and emotional level and died, and then I just thought 'no!' . . . I'm actually defying what the doctors are saying, not because I'm belligerently defiant, but I don't accept that there's only one way to go and that's down and into the ground at this point. [Female, advanced cancer, 2011–2014 study, Australia]

David: . . . you will determine which pathway you go down. Say for an example I did get better, well something miraculous and the cancer has stopped, well there'd be another pathway . . . I might just get sick of the whole deal, I don't know what I'll do, but I don't think I'll give up. I'm not into giving up yet, no it's too early to give up. [Male, advanced cancer, 2011–2014 study, Australia]

There is a wilful disobedience evident in the above excerpts and across many of the interviews and studies explored here. This wilful disobedience is a valued and important facet of living with, and surviving, cancer. But disobedience of what or of whom, and why? Ahmed (2014) states: 'Willfulness involves persistence in the face of having been brought down, where simply to "keep going" or to "keep coming up" is to be stubborn and obstinate. Mere persistence can be an act of disobedience' (p. 2). This is the case in the context of cancer. There is disobedience in relation to the medic, the body, the diagnosis, the clinical knowledge. Just as fear was a prominent feature of the interviewees' accounts, so too was there wilfulness, obstinate determination and rejection of the claims of others to know. In many cases, disobedience was aimed at biomedical figures, and in turn, exploration of complementary and alternative medicine to explore survivorship 'alternatives'. This in turn raised a new set of structures and normative constructs which are worthy of considerable exploration and reflection.

On optimism and complementary medicine

A common strategy of survivorship was the pursuit of complementary and alternative (CAM) medicines to seek healing beyond biomedicine. Often, as a result of the 'terminal prognosis', participants would seek out help from 'alternative' practitioners who would (from many of the patients' perspectives) provide a sense of hope and new possibilities that biomedicine was perceived to disallow (the possibility of healing, the possibility of 'doing something'). In embracing advanced cancer patients – often those deemed futile from an oncological perspective – CAM practitioners capture many of the estranged subjects of biomedicine. Advanced cancer patients use CAM prolifically and there are important reasons for this. Some of these reasons are related to empowerment, and privileging of the subject (rather than the object – disease) in CAM, the de-centring of disease, and the integration of personhood. Engagement with CAM practitioners offered these participants renewed hope, which often became the articulation of wilfulness, the resistance to (biomedical) authority (and acceptance of new forms of authority). CAM practices, as recounted by the participants themselves, drew on their own sense of embodied knowing and intuitive sense of what was required to prevail over their cancer. One of the ways in which we explored this dynamic was to ask some participants to fill in a one-month diary documenting their experiences of living with cancer, using CAM, and the importance for survivorship therein. This diary technique provides an interesting temporal view of the affective dimensions of affliction, and the importance of CAM practices in encouraging what is often discouraged in biomedical encounters (a focus on self and healing).

Below, Theodore documents his engagement with CAM over the month and his disdain for 'bad news' from biomedical practitioners, and 'supportive news' from his CAM practitioner:

Theodore's Diary [2004–2005, United Kingdom]
Day 1: [Theodore lists a substantial dietary and supplement regimen costing over £2000 a month, including daily caffeine enemas] Although it seems like a lot to be taking, it is fairly easy to regulate and really gives me the feeling like I am actively doing something every day. In addition to the pills, I also

try to do a coffee enema every day . . . I feel well in myself and have had neither positive nor negative thoughts.

Day 2: I woke up feeling depressed but after I went round to a friend's house and had a nice chat, I felt much better. Then I received a phone call from [CAM practitioner] who told me he could see a definite improvement in my lymph. I went to bed feeling very positive.

Day 9: I am having a CT scan on the seventeenth of this month. I know that the results will look worse than my first CT scan. The doctors will stress upon me how important it is to have chemo. I do not want to hear how important it is to have chemo. I do not want to hear that as it will cast doubt and fear into my mind and it is important to stay positive . . . What a crazy world we try to live in [sic].

Day 17: A CT scan at the hospital today. Spoke to the nurse who was very supportive of my alternative approach. That's the kind of attitude I want from the doctors – not denouncing the unknown . . . At the end of yoga today, I asked the instructor if there were any exercises I could do that stimulated lymph flow. He told me some. I told him why I wanted to do this and cried. When I got home I cried again, like when I first found the lump and had to tell people I cried. It was nice to let go of some emotion.

Diary entries missing for a couple of days . . .

Day 24: Chatted with [my friend] today. I told [my friend] I found it difficult to keep motivated as I feel so well. Sometimes I have to remind myself that I'm ill, sometimes I slack off a bit for a few days, don't do enemas, don't lymphasise, etc . . . However, I do always take my supplements.

The above diary excerpts illustrate a range of important dynamics related to CAM and cancer survivorship. We can see the value of Theodore's self-care and self-healing activities, but in turn the difficulties of actualising this regimen on a day-to-day basis. He recounts the unhelpfulness of negative feedback from biomedical professionals, but in turn, the difficulties of maintaining his own positivity (amidst doubt and fear) in the fact of illness and his challenging prognosis. His diary reveals the tensions around self-discipline in the context of healing and survivorship, and the internalisation of individual responsibility in order to achieve recovery. Whilst this may be useful for many people – and certainly at points it was for Theodore – and we certainly do not discount the liberatory potential – it also offers new forms of reduction to the subject. After a sense of estrangement from biomedicine, and emerging from the spectre of futility, the person becomes entangled with another set of logics; another series of normative understandings of subject versus object. The problematic nature of these new reductionisms were reflected in participants' accounts of the 'dark side' of CAM and the affective conundrums that participants found themselves struggling with. This including feeling the positivity 'dripping away', feeling forced to 'be vigilant', feeling 'forced into healing', and resisting the pressure to 'be good':

Audrey: For me, I suppose positivity allows me to help myself. So helping myself is a cure for cancer, that's how I receive it. Because I know that if you're not positive, you can feel it, you know. It's acidic in your belly and everything. So that's how I think . . . take the negativity out of your body . . . it's very hard. It's a challenge every day because there are times I cry. No one sees it, but I cry, you know? I cry because what more can I do? It's a challenge every day . . . You have to just be vigilant. [Female, advanced cancer, 2006–2007, Australia]

Delilah: I tend not to get desperate about things. I've gotta think positive and . . . [pauses and thinks for a while] I think that people who have to think positive, that deep down they're not. The fact that they've gotta force themselves to be positive, means that consciously they're being positive but subconsciously . . . it just drips away. [Female, advanced cancer, 2006–2007, Australia]

Constance: Um . . . to be honest in a lot of cases alternative medicine seems too hard. To, for instance, change diet drastically, um yeah, it's hard with food . . . the thought of eating horrible food really puts me off and I don't think I could go vegetarian . . . to maintain the self-discipline and *be good* all the time. [Female, breast cancer, 2006–2007, Australia; emphasis added]

While the interviews touched on the 'back stage' of self-healing, attempts at transcending affliction and the new 'gurus of survivorship', the potential for cruelty within this sphere was palpable in some of the participants' diaries. One British participant, in particular, considered the pernicious potential of notions of will, self-healing and transcending affliction. This participant, Richard, was struggling with advanced cancer, and had been told by his doctors that he had very little time to live. He decided, with his wife, to embark on a strict regimen of self-healing, involving a wide range of extreme dietary measures. This regimen occupied most of his and his wife's time. He was committed to finding a cure for his cancer. In the interview prior to the diary, Richard was highly motivated, driven to self-care and healing, and determined to 'beat it'. His diary starts with a consultation with a CAM therapist and ends with his death:

Richard's Diary [2004–2005, United Kingdom]:
Day 9: Attended [CAM practitioner's] consulting room . . . We learned more about the Gerson [diet].[4] There are three doctors in the UK who have received Gerson training and who claim Gerson credentials but they have their own interpretation. For me, this is confusing and part of medical politics and ego. He [CAM practitioner] talked quite knowingly about the treatment but when I asked him to point out the injection site [for the treatment] on my buttocks, he was not certain . . . He suggested I take two or three juices a day plus a coffee enema until we geared up for the full treatment.

    Day 13: I slept indifferently despite the visualisation described on the Bristol tape of a healing blue light falling on me. Probably my visualisation needs to be improved since I do not produce a clear mental picture but rather a vague adumbrated picture.

Day 14: Visited [doctor's name] who is very sympathetic and warns me not to be so ardent in self-denial, but to listen to my body's requirements.

Day 15: [6am] Started to prepare carrots and apples for the day's juicing . . . I time the procedure to be about three hours.

Day 20: [Support group leader] came to see me after a session. I asked her why they were so against me using the Gerson Therapy. She explained that it is a very demanding and time-consuming therapy and the clinic did not consider it wise at our age . . . This was a very valid point. I think that whilst I have made a critical change it will be best all round [to change to something else] and give us a quality of life together that Gerson could ruin.

Day 22: We have changed course to a less severe therapy therefore more suited to our age.

Admitted to hospital due to infection.

Day 23: I'm awake at 4 am. I have resolve to attempt to modify my diet and exercise more as a self-help therapy. Life is difficult, though now I'm on steroids and I don't know how to balance diet, rest, exercise . . . I am informed that a special bed will be delivered sometime tonight to relieve my sores. I have been thinking of sitting in the chair all night with a blanket around me.

The notes directly above are the last Alan wrote in this diary. Four weeks later, he died at 7:30 am. His wife delivered the diary to Alex Broom and gave a follow-up interview.

The story above is not uncommon in the context of advanced cancer. Some may argue that indeed, his story was a positive one; an ending filled with determination, resistance and the illustration of strength of will. We do not discount such readings. However, the suffering he also experienced – and that of many of the other participants who recounted the underlying, latent sufferings – emerged from a dynamic of reductive self-healing and sense of agency. Lauren Berlant's (2011) concept of cruel optimism rings true here in terms of how some alternative health movements carry normative and moral constructs that can perpetuate and even enhance suffering for cancer patients and those at the end of their life. This re-imaging of the subject-as-agent rather than diseased person, creates the sense, as Berlant (2011) outlines, that being dutiful will indeed result in what one deserves.

While the focus of self-care, self-healing and even self-responsibility in the context of wellness, survivorship and recovery has created an agentive turn within the context of terminal illness (Harrington, 2008), it also offers up new normativities, moral obligations and in some contexts, enhanced individual and family suffering. This is particularly evident in contexts whereby patients with advanced cancer are unable to fulfil their desire to limit or transcend their disease. The focus on the person as agent of change introduces various problematics, including the drive towards self-responsibility, the neoliberal turn towards self-governance, and even a crisis of the self for many whose conditions 'act differently'. The underlying assumption is that health may be part of the person, that illness may be a product of our self (think holistic sickening), offering something as normative and constraining as the focus on external solutions and/or prognostic futility

(Harrington, 2008). Rampant individualism, perceived self-efficacy and devolving responsibility to the individual can have unintended side-effects; and produce suffering in the context of cancer (Illouz, 2007). Through the producing of new disciplinary devices and pathological ontologies (e.g. 'survival-through-character', 'health-through-discipline', 'survivorship-as-individual-heroism') (Stacey, 1997), this sociality of survivorship is *done* rather than *is*, and is heavily embedded in relational dynamics, often with close family and friends surrounding cancer patients.

Survival in relation

In a final reflection on some of the key dimensions of contemporary cancer survivorship, we note that there is a moral economy to survivorship, with its toolkit resulting in what Wetherell (2012) describes as 'circulating affect' – what people themselves often experience as waves of feeling; the collective feeling of the need to survive and to prevail. Cancer as a field is so often imbued with ideas about injustice and untimeliness, and such ideas function to mobilise people who surround those living with or dying from cancer. This creates a moral economy of illness and care, resting on notions of justice for the ill and care for the vulnerable but also the expectation of character in the face of adversity. Survivorship practices are bound to the expectations around how one *should* and *can* act in relation to it. This often sat in stark contrast to the internal worlds of many of the participants, who often suppressed their emotions as they sought to manage the emotions and desires of their significant others. The 'circulating affect' of survivorship was embedded in understandings about what is right and good, and offered a cultural salve to the notion of affliction and dying as unjust and untimely (regardless of the context and conditions of affliction):

Alan: Well, I'm trying to keep a level head. Not to allow myself to get into any form of depressed state of mind. And yeah, be as positive as possible . . . I often thought that if you didn't really care about your family, it'd be a lot easier on everybody when these sort of things arise. [Male, advanced cancer, 2011–2014 Study, Australia]

Annie: I don't talk about the end . . . he [husband] can't cope with that, because he feels that if anything happens to me, that's the end of his life as well . . . So we haven't progressed, we will have to further down the track. But at this point in time, there's no need to, because I'm well. [2011–2014, Australia]

Duncan: . . . I've got an 11-year-old son, as well. I told him I'm going to get better, which was one of my main drivers of, 'I can't die now. Can't die yet.' . . . We had to [talk like that]. I couldn't like [say], 'This thing's eating me away, I'm going to die.' [So] I didn't. [Male, advanced cancer, 2011–2014, Australia]

The 'circulating' feelings around cancer, and the need to prevail, were persistent in the participants' accounts. According to Blackman (2007/08), affective transmission is 'never simply something one "catches" but rather a process that one is "caught up" in' (p. 29). Furthermore, Blackman (2007/08) argues that the complexity of affective transmission is 'revealed through the linkages and connections of the body to other practices, techniques, bodies (human and non-human), energies, judgments, inscriptions and so forth that are relationally embodied' (p. 29). This is the case with cancer survivorship. Many of the participants felt 'lost' in the circulating feelings around cancer. Below, a participant talks about feeling like 'public property' in her battle with cancer, as those around her attempted to manager her life and lifestyle:

Kate: I disagree with the Cancer Council actually, the Cancer Council is inclined to want you to go out there, pin your pink lady on your chest, and shout to the world 'hey, look at me, I have cancer, I have breast cancer.' I don't agree with that. I believe you share it with your closest friends or whoever you want to talk to, but you don't necessarily go out there and shout it to the world. Because the moment you do that . . . [t]wo things happen: you become public property and the second thing is that caring, well-meaning friends tend to want to look after you and *change your lifestyle*. And I think you've got to make those decisions yourself. [emphasis added] [Female, cancer, Australia]

One can see from Kate's excerpt the ways in which the structures around cancer, the moralities, normativities and ethics of practice, bind subjects to particular positions (as survivor, as one who prevails, as a battler). It is interesting to consider how these interplay with the affective. As Blackman (2007/08) notes, problems arise when we 'either reify emotionality as a set of practices of the self or are directed to moments of happiness which just seem to arrive' (p. 29). Similarly, in the context of cancer, the very reception of the disease intersects with its experience. Kate restricts her engagement with others, and their capacity to input into her illness, due to an acute sense of being entrapped in a set of expectations. The well-meaningness is and *feels* estranged from the 'realities' of living with cancer (which incorporates feelings of dread, unhealthiness, hopelessness and 'giving up', as well as hope, enthusiasm, optimism). What these narratives illustrate is an acute awareness of the moral production of the subject, and the price of revealing 'true feelings' given the moral economic of illness and care.

Conclusion

This chapter has explored a (deliberately) mixed series of emotions and practices in and around cancer survivorship. Cancer survivorship has been chosen because illness, suffering and care is a messy arena; and one in which a wide range of logics, discourses and 'players' feed into the negotiation of survival. It is not that we cannot participate in survivorship, illustrating our (free) will and agency, but it is that other *things* shape our moves, inflect our choices and colour our view of the field. In this way, the affective dimensions of surviving *with* cancer encompass and articulate the things that settle on us throughout the experience of affliction, and for some, during the dying process. As we saw in the participant's accounts of being told 'you're terminal', people often resist this clinical spectre, demanding alternative positions, and willing the opportunity to prevail over their disease. Such desires are an assemblage of cultural discourse, social norms, and personal agency. Yet, underlying survivorship practices are distinctly *fearful relations* and the (often cascading) experience of *restlessness* (embodied, somatic, existential, social). These affective responses, and others not explored here, articulate an uneasiness with, and even estrangement from, the dominant construction of cancer survivorship, or indeed, dying well. Thus, there is, often underneath the surface of things, much wondering why suffering and stoicism should prevail. There is a concurrent desire to be the person others want and to meet expectations of self and others. There is also a series of wonderings regarding the purpose, and even the cruelty, of resilience.

Furthermore, a wilful disobedience is evident in the accounts presented above. Often reflected in sharp movement beyond biomedicine, participants resisted almost all parts of the/ir assemblage (body-mind-world-technology and so forth). Often the very forms of resistance they embarked on held new normative qualities, offering similarly potent scripts – this time of self, rather than medicine – to secure their future, to overcome their affliction, and to delay their mortality. This produced a new but still problematic series of scripts which in turn settle on subjects, and interplay with circulating cultural discourses around the self, individualisation, character and agentive potentiality (Illouz, 2007). Essentially, we have sought to present survivorship as a form of sociality; and one that operates at (and secures) the boundaries of things, groups, professions, technologies and discourses. Survivorship is also wrapped up in complex kinship relations and the moral economy of care. That is, desire and hope, hopelessness, resignation, dread each reflect the existence and potency of permissive moral boundaries.

It is worth pointing out, as Wetherell does (2012), that the idea of affective circulation that settles on subjects is problematic. A similar concern may operate in the sphere of survivorship. This 'settling on' 'implies that affect is an ethereal, floating entity, simply "landing" on people' (Wetherell, 2012, p. 141). Wetherell (2012) prefers, as do we, to consider affective practice as something 'encountered as a pre-existing given . . . as though we are entering a 'zone' or an 'atmosphere'. . . that is actively created and needs work to sustain' (p. 142). Such is the case with survivorship. In turn, survivorship illustrates the permeability of bodies and minds, by binding subjects together (see Ahmed, 2004b) – often families, friends, communities and healthcare workers. The 'feelings' of, in and around, survivorship – fear, dread, hope, restlessness, wilfulness exemplify what Ahmed (2004a) describes as the

> rippling effect of emotions; they move sideways (through 'sticky' associations between signs, figures, and objects) as well as backward (repression

always leaves its trace in the present,– hence 'what sticks' is also bound up with the 'absent presence' of historicity).

(p. 120)

The surviving subject can thus be viewed as conceived through 'settlement' by Ahmed (2004a), even if the settlement is in fact constrained by the contours of the subject. From Ahmed's position, 'the subject' is simply one nodal point in the economy, rather than its origin and destination. This is, in turn, a useful way of thinking about survivorship and all its complex affective dimensions. What this means is that the individual and collective are joined, enmeshed, and in turn do not determine one another – they operate *in relation.* In this sense, and again following Ahmed (2004a), the 'cancer survivor' comes into being through its very alignment with (or estrangement from) these collective emotions. In thinking about the emotions circulating survivorship, it is useful to remind ourselves of these relational dynamics:

> Any particular instance of the circulation of affect, whether occurring in consulting rooms, parliamentary committees, football stadiums or in the message boards of the Internet, involves understanding a raft of processes: body capacities to re-enact the actions of others; the developmental infrastructure of inter-subjectivity; the power of words; the affective–discursive genres personal and social histories provide which channel communal affect; inter-subjective negotiations; consideration of the cultural and social limits on identification and empathy; and exploration of practices of authorisation, legitimation and resistance, not to mention analyses of the containing institutions, spaces and media of circulation.

(p. 142)

Similarly, this is pertinent to the field of survivorship and the accounts provided by the participants. If we view survivorship in terms of the circulation of affect, we must acknowledge somatic capabilities; histories of success and failure; inter-subjective encounters; the conditions of care; and the role of abjection in illness and dying. We seek not to diminish forms of innovation or the desire to transcend affliction. Rather, we seek to embed practice in recognition of (often competing) demands, pressures, interests, agendas and the normative. We seek to uncover those factors that might enhance personal suffering and even increase the likelihood of problematic deaths. Emotions therein are critical as they are often conceived in isolated, individualised terms, particularly from a medical perspective. Such terms include 'hopeful', 'strong', 'realistic' and 'accepting'. Conversely, we argue that affect in survivorship is a relation, and treating it as individualised will perpetuate and produce suffering for those living with and dying from cancer.

Notes

1 National bodies for representing and espousing survivorship are ubiquitous in most, if not all, OECD nations, and increasingly, in non-OECD contexts. For examples, see

the Australian Cancer Survivorship Centre (www.petermac.org/about-us/australian-cancer-survivorship-centre), the National Centre for Cancer Survivorship (https://nccs.org.au/), the National Cancer Institute (www.cancer.gov/about-cancer/coping/survivorship) and the Indian Cancer Society (www.indiancancersociety.org/what-do-we-do/rehabilitation.aspx). Whilst most are focused on potentially curable patients and patients who have been cured, their discursive practices permeate disease contexts.

2 Dr John MacArtney assisted with the 2011–2014 (Australia, interview-based) study and Dr Katherine Kenny assisted with the 2015–present (Australia, interview-based). Alex Broom led the 2004–2005 (UK, diary-based) and 2006–2007 (Australia, interview-based) studies alone.

3 We recognise that terminal restlessness, and the therapeutic approaches to this condition, can be an important part of end of life care (see for instance www.pharmaceutical-journal.com/learning/learning-article/dealing-with-the-dying-patient-treatment-of-terminal-restlessness-and-agitation/11119466.article). There is, however, also a need to consider what lies within such practices of medicalisation, and how forms of sedation or pharmaceutical solutions to the agitation of dying, may also act as a panacea for some of the existential, inter-nodal complexities of facing human mortality.

4 The Gerson Diet involves strict diet, dietary supplements, and enemas. The biomedical community largely opposes the claims made on behalf of this diet, and indeed, there is no existing data to prove or disprove those claims (see www.cancer.gov/about-cancer/treatment/cam/patient/gerson-pdq). The Gerson Diet thus presents as a considerable site of controversy and costs a large amount of money to embark on. Often, it is combined with other forms of self-care, including meditation. For further information, see http://gerson.org/gerpress/the-gerson-therapy/.

References

Ahmed, S. (2014). *Willful Subjects*. Durham, NC and London: Duke University Press.

Ahmed, S. (2004a). Affective economies. *Social Text*, *79*, 22(2), pp. 117–139.

Ahmed, S. (2004b). Collective feelings: or, the impressions left by others. *Theory, Culture & Society*, 21, pp. 25–42.

Berlant, L. G. (2011). *Cruel Optimism*. Durham, NC: Duke University Press.

Blackman, L. (2007/2008). Is happiness contagious? *New Formations*, 63, pp. 15–31.

Blackman, L. (2008). *The Body: The Key Concepts*. Oxford, New York: Berg.

Blackman, L. & Venn, C. (2010) Affect. *Body and Society*, 16(1), pp. 7–28.

Broom, A. (2015) Dying: A Social Perspective on the End of Life. London and New York: Routledge; and Farnham: Ashgate.

Broom, A., & Tovey, P. (2007). Therapeutic Pluralism? Evidence, power and legitimacy in UK cancer services. *Sociology of Health and Illness*, 29(1), pp. 551–569.

Broom, A. & Tovey, P. (2008a). Exploring the temporal dimension in cancer patients' experiences of non-biomedical therapeutics. *Qualitative Health Research*, 18(12), pp. 1650–1661.

Broom, A. & Tovey, P. (2008b). *Therapeutic Pluralism: Exploring the Experiences of Cancer Patients and Professionals*. London & New York: Routledge.

Broom, A. & Cavenagh, J. (2011). On the meanings and experiences of living and dying in a hospice. *Health: An Interdisciplinary Journal for the Social Study of Health, Illness and Medicine*, 15(1), pp. 96–111.

Broom, A. & Kirby, E. (2013). The end of life and the family: Hospice patients' views on dying as relational. *Sociology of Health and Illness*, 35(4), pp. 499–513.

Broom, A., Kirby, E., Good, P., Wootton, J. & Adams, J. (2013). The art of letting go: Referral to palliative care and its discontents. *Social Science and Medicine,* 78, pp. 9–16.

Broom, A., Kirby, E., Kenny, K., MacArtney, J., Good, P. (2016). Moral ambivalence and informal care for the dying. *The Sociological Review,* DOI: 10. 1111/1467-954X.12400.

Burke, A. L., Diamond, P. L., Hulbert, J., Yeatman, J. & Farr, E. A. (1991). Terminal restlessness – its management and the role of midazolam. *The Medical Journal of Australia,* 155(7), pp. 485–487.

Dragojlovic, A & Broom, A. (2017). *Bodies and Suffering: Emotions and Relations of Care.* London & New York: Routledge.

Frank, A. W. (2002). *At the Will of the Body: Reflections on Illness.* Boston, MA: Houghton Mifflin.

Harrington, A. (2008). *The Cure Within: A History of Mind-Body Medicine.* London: W. W. Norton & Co.

Illouz, E. (2007). *Cold Intimacies: The Making of Emotional Capitalism.* Cambridge: Polity Press.

Illouz, E. (2008). *Saving the Modern Soul.* Berkeley, CA: University of California Press.

Probyn, E. (2004). Everyday shame. *Cultural Studies,* 18(2/3), pp. 328–349.

Sointu, E. (2015). Discourse, affect and affliction. *The Sociological Review,* 64, pp. 312–328.

Stacey, J. (1997). *Teratologies: A Cultural Study of Cancer.* London: Routledge.

Steinberg, D. (2015). The bad patient: Estranged subjects of the cancer culture. *Body and Society,* 21(3), pp. 115–143.

Wetherell, M. (2012). *Affect and Emotion: A New Social Science Understanding.* London: Sage.

White, C., McCann, M. A. & Jackson, N. (2007). First do no harm . . . terminal restlessness or drug-induced delirium. *Journal of Palliative Medicine,* 10(2), pp. 345–351.

Conclusion
Suffering and caring assemblages

Introduction

In this book, we have sought to interrogate and critique dominant and pervasive notions of suffering as located in, and contained by the individual human body. This has involved critically exploring what it means to 'suffer' across different bodies, relations and social contexts. We do not present our 'cases' as being exhaustive or somehow capturing all the undulations of suffering. Rather, these cases offer (often disruptive) insights into the lived experience of suffering, and the importance of embedding our conceptions of suffering in the everyday. The empirical sites and lived experiences on which our analysis is based urge us not to approach suffering through the reductive, binary logic that positions suffering and illness in fundamental opposition to other states of being, such as health, wellness, contentment, acceptance and happiness. Such normative forces run deep across the chapters, and warrant considerable disruption and critique. We have argued for suffering to be understood through the lens of the 'affective assemblages' – as 'made up by' bodies, discourses, practices and technologies. What this means is that often we do not see all the parts of things; and that we are not aware of the contributors to a moment, a situation or an environment.

Most importantly, in order to make sense of suffering, we have often separated things that are inseparable (e.g. feelings, bodies, discourses). Our aim has been to reconnect these 'things', to reveal enduring connectivities, and to illustrate the fallacies of reductive ideas around, and practices of valorisation in relation to, *individual* suffering. Similarly, we have sought to problematise relations of care across peoples and places. One cannot and *should not* explore suffering as a social relation without understanding the practice, experience and normativity of care and care*giving*. Most importantly, we have sought to understand the limitations of ideas about care as being about gift and exchange – that is, as being a virtuous, ethical practice.

Throughout the book, we have thus sought to critique care and caregiving as being conceived of in thoroughly one dimensional terms; as far too often being conflated with positive forms of affect, and as producing (or being a crucial element of) happy, harmonious relationships. Rather, we have argued that relations of care need to be approached as assemblages of affective intensities of attention, love, compassion, tensions, discrepancies, contradictions, disappointment, loss, sadness, and (at times) psychological and physical harm. In sum, we have sought to reconnect suffering and care, analysing care as not always a solution to suffering (or part of its amelioration), but rather as an actor in the origin, character and perpetuation of suffering. In other words, we have approached care as being a site of suffering in and of itself.

We have explored how studies of neoliberalism convincingly argue that the normalisation of everyday suffering has actually been forged through the persistent production of desire to achieve successful, happy lives that are devoid of suffering. In *Cruel Optimism*, Lauren Berlant (2011, p. 2) argues that relations of cruel optimism is where 'something you desire is actually an obstacle to your flourishing'. Berlant charts how people's attachments to fantasies of a 'good life' overlook those forces of liberal-capitalist societies that are not allowing them to achieve such a life. Her textual analysis reveals affective responses in Euro-American societies where precarity and crisis have become quotidian. While our analysis is in many respects inspired by Berlant's insights, our empirical research has urged us to direct our analytical lens towards the shifting continuum of affective forces that flow between, through and alongside a wider range of emotions; and to attend to the messiness of everyday life (Ahmed, 2010). Our empirical material has cautioned us against the assertion that certain desires are detrimental to a subject's flourishing, and it has encouraged us to pay attention to the shifting continuum between flourishing and demise. More specifically, we have paid particular attention to how engagements with negative and unhappy forms of affect – loss, unhappiness, depression, anxieties, failure and rage – might provide productive sources of potential for ontological transformation. While we acknowledge how suffering has been normalised under neoliberalism, we argue for the necessity of engaging with subjective articulation of affective forces, as this allows us to attend to the complexities of everyday life, to the controversial and the unexpected. Our analytical attention to the detailed empirical material has demonstrated a need for queering the affective dimensions of suffering and relations of care. By this, we mean problematising the binary regimes of health and illness, mind and the body, suffering and happiness from which normative visions about suffering and care emanate.

The practice of queering is focused on unsettling the normative, and emerges from queer theory. The emergence of queer theory in the early 1990s was driven by a poststructuralist, intersectional and transnational understanding of gender, sexuality and social norms, and having the unsettling of the normative, as its core, driving force (e.g. Berlant & Warner, 1995; De Lauretis, 1991; Edelman, 2004; Eng et al., 2005; Muñoz, 1999; Sedgwick, 1993). Given its history, queerness and queer theory is most often associated with sexuality and gender identity, in particular sexual practices and identities that point towards the shifting and unstable nature of identities that have been conceived of as counter-hegemonic. While we have not focused specifically on matters relating to sexual and gender identity, our analysis has been invested in queering the categories of embodiment, suffering, care and care relations.[1] Here, as with Michael Warner (1991, p. xiii), we are interested in the regulatory mechanisms (associated with individuals, families, nations) and their counter-hegemonic possibilities.

In seeking to better conceptualise suffering, we also have gathered together some important conceptual tools, and theoretical insights that are well-developed in the literature, but hitherto had not been brought together. In particular, we have focused in on *what assemblages do* (Deleuze & Guattari, 1987, p. 257), and have approached each of the contexts described in the previous chapters as being reflective of what Lisa Blackman refers to as 'brain-body-world entanglements' (Blackman, 2012, p. 1). That is, we have aimed to locate and reveal connections that have been so often concealed by the attempts to categorise and make sense of suffering and relations of care therein. This has allowed us to attend to the body and embodiment not as static but in a process of continual change and becoming, demonstrating that an analysis of suffering that only focuses on the individual subject or presumes that suffering only belongs to the interiority of the human being would be limiting and counterproductive. We have demonstrated how different bodies, technologies, discourses, practices and performances are constitutive elements of affective assemblages of suffering and the moral economy of caring. We have explored how caring relations are underpinned by complex moralities and forms of obligation that circulate around suffering, care and expectations for 'recovery'. We have explored how moral and ethical *responses to* suffering are experienced, contested, negotiated and institutionalised. The insights provided by our approach aim to challenge dichotomous understanding of suffering and happiness, mind and body, nature and culture, health and illness.

How might we further considering queering suffering and caring relations? We have seen in Chapter 1 that, while professionalism can denote dissociation and detachment, actors/clinical unsettle such strategies and boundaries, suffering in relation, and sharing in the bodily and emotional trauma of the disease. We focused on cancer, and particularly, on doctors and nurses who work with patients in the advanced stages of this disease.

In Chapter 2, we illustrated how emotions deny the normative, offering dread, disgust and abandonment into the mix of supposedly positive associations with 'care' at the end of life. In Chapter 4, we explored how the adult adoptees support group *For Adoptees* has intentionally mobilised affective politics to evoke feelings of discontent, pain, anger, racialisation and marginalisation in order to affectively problematise the pathologisation of adoptees' emotions. These practices directly challenge the widespread therapy cultures emphasis on evoking and producing happy modes of affect such as calmness, balance and contentment.

Similarly, in Chapter 5, we examined a Family Constellation Therapy session for adult adoptees that mobilised what we refer to as the practice of radical affectivity – an intensive, mutual healing sessions that employs performative re-enactments of extreme suffering seeking subjective transformation without the promise of a 'happy end' (in other words, the therapy session does not promise that well-being and happiness will ensue). Each of these sites disrupt existing ideas about who is suffering, and what care is and means, indicating the importance of queering normative understanding of care (as always producing harmonious relations) and suffering (as coming from, and being contained only within a singular human body).

The need for queering of categories of care and caring relations emerged poignantly in Chapter 3, where we ethnographically explored how a one-dimensional understanding of care (parents caring for children) is insufficient when analysing tension-ridden and often psychologically and physically harmful practices within the family in the context of historical violence and family secrecy about biological relatedness of children fathered by enemy soldiers. In Chapter 4, we explored how the everyday racialisation of non-white adoptees growing up in white families and the society that imagines itself as white (the Netherlands), seems to have been a common experience for adult adoptees who were members of the *For Adoptees* group. As part of this investigation, we found that the caring practices of an adoptee's extended family and their social network were often racialised.

Moving atmospheres: the circulation of suffering

One of the key contributions we see this book as making is reimagining and reconfiguring suffering as necessarily circulating, as moving across persons, communities, generations and as certainly not standing still (nor inside an individual person). Many of the categories that we rely on heavily in social life contribute to the concealment of this affective circulation. The idea of the 'professional carer', the idea of the 'next generation', the idea of 'the living' and 'the dying' are replete with binaries which do not hold up in practice. These ideas deny the shifting nature of suffering. That is, suffering is not neatly located where it often might be presumed to be; it moves, it lies underneath, it moves across the – sometimes in more or less obvious forms. There is the sense that suffering may only *become* when it is acknowledged, when it is recognised, and when pervasive categories are contested. In this way suffering in fact *is* how we consider it, how we *treat* it, and how we recognise it. By making assumptions about suffering and what it can be, we only recognise 'suffering' within the assumed, dominant categories of the given cultural milieu. By disrupting the borders between things (as we have done here), we can see how in fact we all have a shared (albeit varied) stake in suffering, and that suffering is constantly *in* circulation. We can also see that suffering does not stop because certain actors or stakeholders die or are no longer 'present'. While the assemblage of life, suffering and care may change, trauma, distress and suffering will exist within *and* beyond; within *and* without – they do not end neatly, as is often assumed. In this way, a dying person's experience of suffering occurs in relation to other people and factors, and this is how it moves with and across people, whether these are professional carers, family members, or partners.

In turn, we have emphasised that suffering is not bound by time. Moments in time, and those of other generations, continue to haunt the present, making their presence known, and refusing to stay 'in the past'. Suffering is thus not bound by the conditions of professional labour or by ideas about timely or untimely deaths; it does not abide by such rules governing bodies and emotions. Finally, we have posited that people feel things (often 'in their bodies'), regardless of the normative, and regardless of the categorisations of things. In a close examination of suffering, we can unsettle the rules of the game; and show that people suffer things they are not supposed to; and that they do not care (or do care) for things that they are supposed to.

Our study suggests that it is important to explore the micro, the everyday of suffering, to dispose of the normative and what conceals things, experiences, feelings and relations. It is insufficient to merely identify that suffering circulates. Rather, as we have done here, research must illustrate the instances of its circulation – the who and what it involves, and the consequences for all those involved in this suffering. It is only by immersing ourselves as researchers in particular sites of suffering that we have been privy to the disruptive relations of suffering and care. We have seen how that which we so often view as normal, acceptable, and necessary is in fact part of the suffering itself. We have shown that normative demands for *being* (a good child, a good professional, a good cancer patient, a compassionate carer) reject the process of *becoming* (a frustrated carer, a hopeless carer, an emotional professional) and thus the very character of suffering-in-relation. The body, as is clearly captured in Blackman's work, becomes a 'surface' whereby the concealed is vividly revealed; with the knowing body expressing what is concealed by (normatively imbued) cognition. The moving atmosphere settles on the body, offering forms of knowing and understanding often in direct contrast to what 'should be'. This moving atmosphere rests on multiple bodies; it is not a singularity but a plurality. How it reveals itself and is revealed, remains contingent and context-specific. Suffering, as it were, is an entanglement; unstable, contingent, affecting and moving.

Sites of suffering for examination in the future

There are a wide range of events, sites, and areas of suffering, as well as particular spheres, which would benefit from further critical exploration. The first is the notion of disaffection, local discontents and the global politics of 'othering'. Much has been written about what is currently occurring in terms of the politics of fear, risk and disaffection, but the current environment is seeing new communities emerging as experiencing suffering. Witness the so-called 'Brexit' vote in the UK/ Europe, and Donald Trump's electoral victory in the US. Both of these moments took place in 2016, and both have (albeit to varying degrees) been articulated as products of the discontent and displacement of (often previously dominant) communities in the new global order (see Quah & Mahbubani, 2016). This discontent and displacement of these communities should be the topic of future research.

The second sphere worthy of investigation is the current global and local environment, and how this environment – or, rather, these environments – are connected with people's lived experience. Here, we refer to how neoliberalism and late modernity are *affecting* the everyday, how we may connect things often not viewed as being connections (feelings, bodies, technologies), and unpack forms of suffering therein. For example, there has been considerable exploration of how people relate to one another in the current cultural milieu, and experiences of anxiety, dislocation and polarisation (among other relations). We suggest focusing on how things are connected, how bodies know things that we (minds) may not seem to understand, and thus how our very ideas about these issues separately belie our experience of the world. Moreover, we suggest focusing on how current technologies and ways of being may shape and be complicit in our lived experiences of suffering (and healing) therein. In the context of medicine, this may mean asking, is treating disease in fact reducing suffering across parts of the person, community, society? In the context of the ever-expanding forced mobility of people across national borders, the question remain how experiences endured during such hardships will affect people subjected to such mobility regimes and their descendants in the future. We argue that future research on the affective dimensions of violence and forced mobility will need to expand on our theorisation of hauntings and transmission of trauma across generations.

Note

1 For the queering of categories and practices that go beyond gender identity and sexuality, see Sullivan and Murray (2009).

References

Ahmed, S. (2010). *The Promise of Happiness*. Durham, NC: Duke University Press.

Berlant, L. G. (2011). *Cruel Optimism*. Durham, NC: Duke University Press.

Berlant, L. & Warner, M. (1995). What does queer theory teach us about X? *PMLA: Publications of the Modern Language Association of America*, 110(3), pp. 343–349.

Blackman, L. (2012). *Immaterial Bodies: Affect, Embodiment, Mediation*. Thousand Oaks, CA: Sage.

De Lauretis, T. (1991). Queer theory: Lesbian and gay sexualities. An introduction. *Differences: A Journal of Feminist Cultural Studies*, 3(2), pp. iii–xviii.

Deleuze, G. & Guattari, F. (1987). *A Thousand Plateaus: Capitalism and Schizophrenia*. London/New York: Continuum.

Edelman, L. (2004). *No Future: Queer Theory and the Death Drive*. Durham, NC: Duke University Press.

Eng, D., Halberstam, J. & Muñoz, J. E. (2005). Introduction: What's queer about queer studies now? *Social Text*, 23(3–4), pp. 1–17.

Muñoz, J. E. (1999). *Disidentifications: Queers of Color and the Performance of Politics*. Minneapolis, MN: University of Minnesota Press.

Quah, D. & Mahbubani, K. (2016). Trump, Brexit and voter discontent. *Bangkok Post*, 16 December, 2016. Available at: www.bangkokpost.com/opinion/opinion/1160785/trump-brexit-and-voter-discontent (Accessed 14 January, 2017).

Sedgwick, E. K. (1993). *Tendencies*. Durham, NC: Duke University Press.

Sullivan, N. & Murray, S., eds. (2009). Somatechnics: Queering the technologisation of bodies. Farnham and Burlington, VT: Ashgate.

Warner, M. (1991). Introduction: Fear of a queer planet. *Social Text*, 29, pp. 3–17.

Index

abandonment 86
Abraham, Nicolas 73
acceptance of dying 46–8
'active treatment,' continuance of 28, 36, 37, 38, 48
adoptees, transnational 86–109; adaptation and assimilation, 87; affection required, 87; attachment disorder as psychopathologisation 87–9; *Bastard Nation Bed Time Stories* 100–3; birthday parties 100–1; as blank slates 92–3; 'disembedded' and 'out of place' bodies 95–100; ethnographic setting 90–2; international adoption agencies 96–7; 'kinning,' 88; pathologisation of 86–9, 93–4; radical affective politics 94–5, 98, 103; 'rooted child' 92–3; scholarship by adoptees, 93; self-transformation 113–4; slavery equated with 94, 95, 96–7; transformation of family life 88–90
'adoption medicine' 86
adoption practices 13, 68–9, 80
affect: bodily 125–8; enhancement or depletion, 127; transmission of 8, 73–4, 98, 148–9
affective assemblages 154; inter-generational suffering as 61–2, 64, 67–8, 74, 77–8, 80–1; secrecy and 62, 68; suffering as 3–6, 21–2
affective entanglements 23
affective intensities 4–5, 22–3, 68, 72, 77, 81, 98–9, 102, 128, 154–5
affective turn 3
agency and choice 7, 8, 147, 149–50
Ahmed, Sara 5, 7, 14, 132, 137, 138; on fear 139–40; generative qualities of affect 4, 22; on wilfulness 142–4, 150–1
ancestors/ancestral field 114, 115, 119
anticipatory grief 24–5, 140

assemblages of suffering 2–4, 154–7; survivorship 6, 134, 138–9. *See also* affective assemblage
assimilation 88, 99
Association of Japanese-Indisch Descendants (JIN) 76–80
atherosclerosis 11
atmosphere, affective 21–2, 97–8, 157–8
attachment disorder 87
Australia 10

'bad patient' 37
Bastard Nation Bed Time Stories 94–5, 100–3
becoming 9, 62, 80–1, 89, 128, 158
being in and being with suffering 6–9
being in car, 21
being in suffering, 21
being with suffering, 21
Bendelow, G. 10–1
bereavement period 21, 43, 56
Bergquist, K. J. S. 93
Berlant, Lauren G. 14, 133–4, 147, 155
biological relatedness 61
biomedical imaginary 5
Blackman, Lisa 4, 9, 11, 63, 103, 126, 134, 141, 149; brain-body-world entanglements 12, 14, 63, 126, 134, 140, 156
bodies: adoptees, psychopathologisation of, 87; disciplining of 2–3; 'disembedded' and 'out of place' 95–100; of health professional, suffering in 27–8, 37; memory incorporated in 63, 67; multiplicity of 10–2; non-white, 87; secrecy and feeling 72–5; of transnational adoptees 95–100
The Body Multiple: Ontology in Medical Practice (Mol) 11
Body & Society 5

For Product Safety Concerns and Information please contact our EU
representative GPSR@taylorandfrancis.com
Taylor & Francis Verlag GmbH, Kaufingerstraße 24, 80331 München, Germany

www.ingramcontent.com/pod-product-compliance
Ingram Content Group UK Ltd.
Pitfield, Milton Keynes, MK11 3LW, UK
UKHW021455080625
459435UK00012B/512